D0251128

# A KINGDOM OF
# TENDER COLORS

Seth Greenland

# A KINGDOM OF TENDER COLORS

A Memoir
of Comedy, Survival, and Love

Europa
*editions*

Europa Editions
214 West 29th Street
New York, N.Y. 10001
www.europaeditions.com
info@europaeditions.com

Library of Congress Cataloging in Publication Data is available
ISBN 978-1-60945-583-5

Greenland, Seth
A Kingdom of Tender Colors

Book design by Emanuele Ragnisco
www.mekkanografici.com

Cover image: © Seth Greenland

Prepress by Grafica Punto Print – Rome

Printed in the USA

# CONTENTS

To Susan, always
To Dr. James Speyer
To Dr. Nicholas Gonzalez (1947-2015)

My own nature, as I am not ashamed to confess frankly,
is unheroic.
—STEFAN ZWEIG

# PROLOGUE

I hold my father's copy of *Mein Kampf* in my hand and wonder if it should be saved, donated, or burned in the backyard. Will the day arrive when I attempt to hack my way through Hitler's turgid opus? Or do I want to observe the look on the face of the clerk at the local donation center when she sees that noxious title? And what was Leo Greenland, husband, father, grandfather, successful advertising executive and generous supporter of multiple charities—some of them Jewish—doing with a paperback edition of *Mein Kampf* anyway? Bequeath, retain or incinerate: Our choices.

We are breaking down Dad's library. His heart gave out six months earlier at ninety-one, and my wife Susan and I have flown east to meet my brother Drew and close down the house. My mother died twenty years earlier and with the eternal absence of both parents the scrim that separates me from death has vanished. Dad was born in the Bronx and my mother in Brooklyn. They ascended high above their social origins and with a well-developed sense of herring-flecked drollery would occasionally refer to themselves as Bix and Brooke.

The bedrooms were easy to pack up; the living room and the den done on autopilot. It would have been easy enough to turn the kitchen into an emotional minefield. There are the beautifully painted dishes my mother shipped from Spain, the ones on which she prepared her signature dish of scallops with feta cheese and tomatoes. The carving knife Dad had wielded so many Thanksgivings or the stained wood tray I had made in elementary school might easily have sent me tumbling down a

Proustian rabbit hole, unable to emerge for hours. These objects resonate, but their emotional power pales compared to that exerted by the books.

In a house of readers, what more than books allows access to the inner lives of its occupants? When a person you love has recently died, there is often an urge to keep them close in some tangible way. With dusty fingers we work our way through libraries of the dead and read their lives, written in volumes about other subjects.

Born to uneducated immigrant parents, Dad was an autodidact (a word he never would have used) whose lifelong search for knowledge and meaning led him on a journey that began with books about marketing and took him from there to the Greek philosophers, particularly Aristotle and Plato. In between, he accumulated a veritable Waldorf salad of titles. There were over a thousand. You can't keep them all.

Bequeath, retain or incinerate. We vow to exorcise sentiment, sort rigorously, keep it moving.

The library is on the second floor of the house, overlooking a frozen lake. No other houses are visible, only ice and bare trees against white sky. When packing our dead father's books on a silent January day, gray winter light flooding in, thoughts of eternity wrestle with the anodyne task at hand. An old bestseller easily drops into the donation pile, but then I am brought up short by a high school yearbook from 1938 and open it to the picture of Dad as an eighteen-year old, his entire life about to unfold, nothing more than a glint in his brown eyes. He looks like my brother—not my brother Drew but a brother of mine in some other dimension, one where we are the same age as our parents and our grandparents and our children and the normal distinctions no longer abide. He is me and I am him. The idea of people you love living on within you no longer seems like such thin gruel.

I decide to keep a leather-bound edition of *Treasure Island*, a book I haven't read since the fourth grade, perhaps because I might read it again, but if I'm being honest, more because it helps me remember that I was once a child and lived with parents who gave me books like that and *The Catcher in the Rye* and *Huckleberry Finn* and to whom I owe gratitude that deepens like the notes of a descending scale on a double bass.

There are histories and biographies, art books, novels, books about golf, classics from antiquity, the entire oeuvre of Ogden Nash, leather-bound volumes both antiquarian and recent, all of them revelatory in one way or another. There are books that my brother and I had given as gifts and we open them to read the inscriptions: "I know if a book has the word 'Jews' or 'Israel' in the title, you will like it. I hope I'm right this time. Love, Seth." In the Alec Guinness memoir *A Blessing In Disguise*, I had written "To Mom, A blessing undisguised." And, of course, I had to stop and stare out the window while I collected myself and thought about all the childhood hours my mother read to me, a book open on her lap as I lay in bed listening.

Turning back to the shelves I pick up a volume of *Remembrance of Things Past*—the Proustian rabbit hole itself!—inscribed in 1938 by my now ninety-year-old Aunt Claire to my paternal grandfather, a four-times married, pathological narcissist from Poland who cut a swathe through the ladies of the Bronx. It is difficult to imagine him having had time for Proust, but it makes me think of my aunt at sixteen, poignantly hoping that her perpetual disappointment of a mostly-absent father might somehow be interested in this book. And then there is this depth charge: an edition of *Now We Are Six* by A.A. Milne, copyright 1927, and inscribed as follows: "To my belove [*sic*] son Leo. Father." When my grandfather abandoned his family in 1928, leaving my grandmother to face the Depression alone with three children, it left my father with an unseen scar. If Dad could be said to have had a primal wound, this was it. To touch the book, a frayed, orange hardback with faded gold lettering, is to hear once again the painful stories he told me about his father, the serial remarriages, the emotional abuse, the years-long estrangement.

Although my parents were not bibliophiles in the traditional sense, every house they occupied had a floor to ceiling wall of books. The first time I ever saw a swastika it glowered at me from Dad's copy of William L. Shirer's *The Rise and Fall of the Third Reich*, shelved near his edition of *Mein Kampf*, cheek-by-jowl with Deborah Lipstadt's *The War on the Jews*. When interested in a subject, he examined it from all angles. I had helped myself to the Shirer years earlier. As for the worthy Lipstadt, it lands in the donation pile.

There is a collection of classics that includes Lucretius, Epictetus and Marcus Aurelius. I have no idea if he read these particular editions, but their contents were manifest in his behavior. He was both an Epicurean and a man who tried to see with the unsurpassed clarity of the Stoics. The art books are a testament to his uxorious nature. My mother was the art lover and they were purchased for her: eclectic volumes of Wyeth, Grandma Moses, El Greco, Monet, Miro, Picasso, Van Gogh, Hopper, Christo, Magritte, Matisse, Garry Winogrand, and Irving Penn. As we sort, all the museum visits come flooding back, my mother's endless quest to make us interested in things besides baseball cards or digging holes in the backyard. Several volumes go into the box I will ship to California.

Three of my Sunday school textbooks have been saved, books I had not laid eyes on in over forty years. One of them contains the following self-penned inscription: "In case of fire, burn this first." I can't imagine either of my parents ever saw it. Their silence in such an event would have been unimaginable. The strange feeling of wanting to excoriate the wisenheimer who scrawled such offensive words overcame me, to remind the little shit of the book burnings that lit Germany in the 1930s, and then, in the kind of psychological jiujitsu that arrives with age, the dissonance of having come to embody the parental position is duly noted. Would I have freaked out if I had discovered my son had done the same? It is difficult to fathom why there are several multivolume collections of humor among Dad's books. My father embodied many qualities when I was young. He was loving, forthright, strong, decisive, and occasionally loud. He was not a teller of jokes. Perhaps the humor anthologies—the S.J. Perelman, the works of Catskills comedian Sam Levenson—were, like Aristotle and Plato, aspirational. His adult life as a propulsive businessman didn't leave much time for hilarity, and I don't recall him laughing that much when I was a child. But judging from his library, it appears as if he wanted to. The Perelman volumes go into the California box.

Books on marketing proliferate, many from the mid-century era, his apotheosis. And next to them a worn paperback of Saul Alinsky's *Rules for Radicals*, so recently a cudgel with which Republicans were trying to thump President Obama. The business books are all placed in the donation pile, the Alinsky set aside. A first edition of an obscure Graham Greene novel, *A Burnt-Out Case*, is a major find, but even though Dad aspired to write fiction when he served in the Army during World War II (we encountered several early efforts as we sorted through his papers), there are not a lot of old novels. There are, however, a great many newer editions of old ones that he had purchased via mail order through something called the Franklin Library. With their gold-lettered leather bindings they have the look of set dressing one would see on a Broadway stage in a production of *The Winslow Boy*. In his Bronx childhood, our essentially fatherless father had somehow learned to ride a horse with an English saddle. Like Gatsby, he had sprung from his platonic conception of himself, and that image required shelves lined with leather volumes. As Drew slips a leather-bound edition of *The Sun Also Rises* into his stack, he remarks that it was as if Dad was filling in an area he had missed when he was trying to get somewhere.

A wonderful oddity is *Zero Mostel Reads A Book*. My parents venerated Zero Mostel, owned several of his signed lithographs, and spoke reverently of having seen him in the American premiere of the Ionesco play *Rhinoceros* in the late fifties. This particular work is nothing more than a rice-paper-wrapped collection of photographs of, yes, Zero Mostel reading a book. I can tell you: Zero Mostel has an awfully expressive face. This made me wonder how many libraries contain copies of both *Zero Mostel Reads A Book* and *Mein Kampf*.

There are books that whisper—from a great distance, their voices barely audible—the quintessence of gone pop culture eras. *Passages* by Gail Sheehy and *Running* by Jim Fixx. A beat-up copy of *All the President's Men*. Titles that were on everyone's lips, books that held the light long enough, and died off early enough, to call forth an entire epoch when their jackets are glimpsed. *Torch Song Trilogy* by Harvey Fierstein, anyone? A one-way ticket to Donationville.

And speaking of plays—my parents were great theatergoers, and although published plays are not represented heavily in the library, the few that are there unleash a cascade of memories: my mother insisting I ask John Gielgud for an autograph (in 1968 when I had no idea who he was), or spending an entire day watching the Royal Shakespeare Company's epic staging of *Nicholas Nickleby* or attending the premiere of *Angels in America* with both of my parents healthy and brimming with life. We donate an omnibus of modern classics, even *No Exit* by Sartre. I hesitate when I sight, eerily, *Da* by the Irish playwright Hugh Leonard, a play about a man haunted by the demanding, irascible, loving ghost of his father. I saw the Broadway production starring Barnard Hughes with my parents in 1976. Dad's copy is with me now.

Some of what was donated: all of the business books and anything having to do with golf. *Good as Gold* by Joseph Heller did not make the cut and neither did Heller's Guillain-Barré memoir that I had mistakenly given Dad as a gift. It was the only time he was incredulous at something I had purchased for him. He didn't do disease. A man of action, he was uninterested in an author's sickbed ruminations. Born on March 4th, his motto—"March forth."

A very short list of what I kept: art books, the *Collected Works of Ogden Nash*, a Bellow novel, *Inside the Third Reich* by Albert Speer (unlike Hitler's opus, my brother assured me, Speer is generally considered to have turned out a first-rate book). And my Sunday school texts. At exorcising sentiment, it turns out, I am a failure.

It takes us two days to finish going through the library. Perhaps it could have been done at a brisker pace, but that would not have allowed unhurried time with our mother and father. We load two cars with the donations and head for a public library in a quiet Connecticut town near where my brother lives. There we fill two bins, each the size of a couple of bathtubs, with our cargo of paper and ink and memory. A woman wanders over to see what we are giving away. The inert pile of books is like an open coffin.

As we drive off I wonder about *mein kampf*. Not the book—that was in the garbage, garlanded with coffee grounds and orange peels—but the struggle, my own struggle, with my father's legacy, with what to keep and what to let go. We are like our parents in ways we cannot imagine, some beguiling and others less so. But we also, even as adults, sometimes consciously embody their qualities. As parents recede in death and memory becomes porous, certain particulars will linger: a favorite melody, the jaunty tilt of a hat, a library. In those details elements of our own identity can be found.

# PART 1
## SCHRODINGER'S CAT

My name is Seth Greenland and I am *not* an alcoholic. Nor am I a drug abuser, sex addict, or overeater. I am not a philanderer, a movie star, or a professional athlete. I am not a politician, captain of industry, or supermodel.

I tell stories.

The spine of this one takes place about twenty-five years ago during a particularly hellish time. Everything I've experienced since then has been refracted through that prism. It was not the particular prism I was hoping for and in the ensuing years I've been trying to make sense of the way its memory has bent the light.

I worry about my lack of standing as a memoirist. I am a novelist and a playwright, but I've made my living writing for television and the movies which is a lunchbox job even when the lunchbox is stuffed with food from Spago. If I didn't earn my keep as a writer, a job many people mistakenly consider interesting, there would be nothing remotely compelling about me. And since I currently live in Los Angeles where if you throw a Xanax tablet you will hit ten of us, there *is* nothing remotely compelling about me.

I am a man who has sex with women. All right—*woman*, singular, if you must know—specifically, my wife who is, incidentally, the only wife I've ever had, leaving me entirely devoid of ex-spouses against whom I could rail in a memoir. I am a garden variety cisgender male married to a cisgender female.

My childhood was ham on Wonder Bread, playground basketball and piano lessons, the New York Yankees, Knicks, and Giants, looking for trouble in nearby woods, running across broad grassy fields, and struggling to stay awake in the public school I attended, all scored to rock and roll music and the tinkling of Good Humor truck bells before that sound became cinematic shorthand for imminent mayhem. The above description might read as overly romantic, but even with some allowance for poetic license, and the requisite golden haze that often casts a luminous glow on any fundamentally positive recollection, and admitting to some minor crimes, broken bones, and being yelled at by the occasional adult, it pretty much accords with reality. My father did not systematically beat me, molest me, or force me to play the viola. He did, however, repeatedly and from early days suggest I become a lawyer which I believe, retrospectively, to be a form of child abuse—just not severe enough to construct a memoir around. My mother was for the most part equally restrained, although she showed an interest in paddle tennis that bordered on the obsessive, only not to the point where it was memoir material. Her emotions would sometimes get the better of her and she would shout and occasionally curse but calm returned soon enough and neither she nor her secret boyfriend killed anyone. In photographs from the 60s she resembles Audrey Hepburn. She never had a secret boyfriend.

During college, I considered taking time off and touring the world, learning new languages and having dangerous adventures in exotic places. Loosening the shackles of expectation. But I didn't. Instead, I graduated in the requisite four years and went to work as a copyboy at the *New York Daily News.* There I met Jimmy Breslin, Pete Hamill, and Liz Smith. They were famous columnists and pleasant to deal with although Ms. Smith did not make eye contact with me the time I arrived at her high-rise apartment to pick up her copy. I wish I could write a raffish book about my exploits with bigtime New York journalists but, to be honest, I encountered each of them only once. Breslin laughed when I called him Mr. Breslin and said "Mistah" in his Queens accent, mocking my formality. He preferred to be called Jimmy. It's a cute detail but would make for a very short memoir. And no one remembers them now.

Back then there was a bar on East 44th Street called Costello's where all the ink-stained reprobates went to get hammered after work. It was noisy and dark and filled with people who read the *Racing Form*. The romantic warp and woof of lives vividly lived, poetically wasted. I wish I got drunk with these people night after night at Costello's. I went there once.

When I published my first novel, I appeared on a panel with an author known to be a former addict. You might say it was his "brand." He informed the audience, who were hanging on his every word because of his ex-junkie gravitas, that he is contractually obligated to mention his former addiction at least once in the course of every public appearance. It was a joke but, really, it wasn't. He has gotten a lot of mileage out of opioids and, not coincidentally, a fine book. I wish I had been an addict.

I have a friend who was a Sandinista. In her tempestuous youth she and her comrades hid out in the Nicaraguan jungle and plotted the overthrow of a brutal dictator. I mention this because she wrote a thrilling memoir about it. I wish I had been a revolutionary. For memoir purposes, it's better than being a junkie.

Because I have written for both television and movies, I have had the opportunity to meet a number of celebrities. I also met Johnny Haymer, the man who played the Catskills comic in *Annie Hall* who wants Woody Allen's character to write gags for him. Johnny Haymer was less dull than most of the celebrities. But does anyone want to read my book-length reflections on Johnny Haymer? Paul Theroux wrote a highly unusual memoir about his tortured relationship with V.S. Naipaul. I had a meeting with Robert De Niro. I wish he was as interesting as V.S. Naipaul, and that we had more than one meeting. Perhaps then our relationship would be tortured and I could write about it. He didn't say much in the meeting. I would have to make a lot of it up because you can't have Robert De Niro playing himself and barely give him any lines. I choose to avoid that ethical quandary.

Still, it is the writer's job to be compelling with the tools at hand.

Every week as a kid, I looked forward to *The Ed Sullivan Show* and my favorite acts were the comedians. My parents were loving but they were not funny. At that time, Dad was particularly not funny. Nor did he exhibit much appreciation for comedy or humor of any kind other than the light verse of Ogden Nash (*Candy is dandy, but liquor is quicker*), whose doggerel style he imitated on those rare occasions when he would attempt to write a poem. Life was not funny to my father, forsaken son of the Bronx who had to scrap for every morsel. He was more comfortable being angry or stern than funny. This would change in later years when he developed a dry sense of humor, but as the forbidding 6'2" authority figure in my life he was distinctly short on the laughs. The comics on the Sullivan show were mostly brisket-fed Jewish men of Dad's generation and the Hennys, Sheckys, and Jackies were the hilarious uncles I wished I had. Their jokes were mostly about banal subjects like airline food or their mothers-in-law but the laughter they provoked was liberating and cathartic. To my father, laughter was anarchic, and not in a good way but in a Mikhail Bakunin let's-abolish-all-government way. It threatened authority and the hierarchical order that decreed who wielded power. Needless to say, I was not encouraged to be funny. As I stumbled from childhood to adolescence, here's how my father usually met my nascent attempts at wit: *Don't be a wiseass.* It was not said in anger, more like a reminder—this thing that you think is amusing will get you nowhere. Although I dutifully tried to take his advice and repress my own anarchic tendencies, laughter was heroin without the needle marks or risk of early death. One of the great benefits of my weed smoking years (approx. 1973–85) was the gale force laughter that would cut through the haze of smoke and jam band music. In a middle-of-the-night café in Berkeley, California, after a twelve-hour drive from Vancouver, there was an epic laughing attack with my brother that went on for at least twenty minutes and might be the closest I've ever come to having seen the face of God. Amazingly, we were not high at the time.

For much of my early life, I internalized Dad's attitude, intended to follow his sober advice and become a lawyer. It's obvious to me now that I would've been a miserable attorney, the kind who wrote scripts for television shows, put them in a drawer (the same one holding the first draft of this memoir for the past ten years), and developed a drinking problem; but growing up in a New York suburb where most of the fathers were doctors, lawyers, or enthusiastic capitalists, it made sense at the time and I held to this plan. While taking the law boards as a senior in college I had a St. Paul-on-the-road-to-Damascus moment in which Jesus told me not to be a lawyer. Not *Jesus* Jesus, of course, but Jesus the metaphor for the tiny part of my brain that understood I was headed toward frustration, disappointment, and self-loathing. Of course, that's where showbusiness landed me, and we'll get to that.

When I graduated from college, my ability to write coherent sentences led to a brief career in journalism and I found myself writing about the New York comedy clubs of the late 1970s, to which I was drawn like a felon to a bank vault. Spending time with comedians, I observed their speech patterns, attitudes,

and philosophies, and began a process of subconsciously inter-
nalizing them. Most of the comics were Jews, but they were not
like the tennis playing Jews among whom I had grown up in
Scarsdale. This community was from Brooklyn, the Bronx, and
Long Island and they had not succumbed to the faux
Protestant Jewish zeitgeist that prevailed in Westchester. A
theory: Jews in the outer boroughs and Long Island were
largely surrounded by other Jews and so remained more insular
where the ones who moved to Westchester found themselves
among upscale Protestants and Catholics and felt greater pressure to keep their heads down and assimilate. Perhaps this is
why Westchester Jews do not as a rule have New York accents.

The Jews I grew up around acted like Episcopalians. Not
these New York City comedy Jews. They rejected the idea of
academic achievement and proficiency at tennis on which I
was raised, were never going to do anything respectable. The
rampant Jewish id was spritzing into a microphone in front of
a roomful of strangers and I was seduced.

It occurred to me that my repressed flair for the funny
could be employed to my benefit. On visits home, I flexed this
newly unfettered skill and family dinners became gladiatorial
venues where I would make my mother roar with laughter
while Dad looked on, stone-faced at this Oedipal threat. I was
performing material but still, it felt good to kill.

If only I were able to do this professionally.

Enter my friend Leonard.

Although fourteen years my senior, Leonard and I were pals
from the moment we spied each other over rails of cocaine—
say hello to 1978—in the den of iniquity that was the basement
of Catch a Rising Star. Turned out we were neighbors downtown and when I moved out of a girlfriend's apartment and
had nowhere to store my tatty possessions Leonard let me park
them at his place. Thin as a pipe cleaner, with an enviable head
of graying hair and the scars of teenage acne partially hidden

by a trim salt and pepper beard, Leonard's easygoing disposition concealed a roiling turbulence. After serving in the Air Force in Japan, he trained as a therapist and was leading a group at the Payne-Whitney Clinic one day when he began to wonder when the therapist was going to arrive and checked himself in. After that it was one oddball New York hustle after another until he unexpectedly found himself writing comedy for a WNBC radio show hosted by his brother. When Leonard hired me to work with him my fate was, as they say, sealed. He was as dysfunctional as any comedy writer I would ever meet—an exceedingly high bar—but I'm not sure I ever laughed more than during my scuffling years in New York when we sprawled in his studio apartment on Prince Street drinking takeout coffee and writing jokes.

"Babe," he would say—it was the name we called each other, deployed to lampoon the cheesy false intimacy of show-business. "Here's a premise—" He pitched a joke, and I would laugh or suggest an adjustment, and then we proceeded to the next bit that needed to be generated. It was almost impossible to believe someone was paying me to do this.

To be a comedy writer was to cultivate a particular sensibility. Everything in life was fair game, a source of material, a potential joke. Nothing off limits. To take something seriously was to betray the whole concept. The font of this, the *sine qua non* was the sainted Lenny Bruce who upon hearing of the Kennedy assassination took the microphone and said, "Poor Vaughn Meader." Meader is one of the great footnotes of nightclub history, a comic whose act consisted of a JFK impression and his comedy album *First Family* had recently reached #1 on the Billboard charts. Bruce's take could not have been more perverse. That many "civilians" would never laugh at a line like that made it even funnier.

*Too hip for the room* was a point of pride.

With my turning pro, years of repression were cast off and

I allowed my mind to go in its disorderly direction. There are people who work in comedy that are always "on" and, while this can be enjoyed in small doses, they become insufferable. For about five minutes I projected that persona but found it ill-suited to my borderline slothful rhythm. Being "on" took too much effort. What I did do was vent ideas that had been suppressed in childhood. The censored remark was unshackled. The id unbound. Want to know what I think? Let me *tell* you. Don't care to know? I'll *still* tell you. And there's going to be a punchline. When I dabbled in therapy and quit after a few sessions, friends asked me why and I said, Because I thought I should be charging a two-drink minimum.

Bada *bing!*

Therapy for someone like me was risible since my response to it was to make the therapist laugh.

Comedy became a way of being in the world, a tactic deployed in reaction to life. A forceful response to stimuli, a defense as powerful as an uppercut. There's an aggression to it, a taking charge that brooks no challenge. It allows an individual to control the interaction whether she is onstage in front of a crowd or in an elevator with one other person. It's the last word. It was a great insight to understand that laughter is involuntary, a form of surrender to the will of the other. I am still so imbued by the comedic sensibility that it feels wrong to make these points and not end with a joke.

I've always loved doctor jokes. Leonard told me this one:

A guy walks into a doctor's office. The doctor says, I have bad news. You have cancer, and you also have Alzheimer's Disease. And the guy says, At least I don't have cancer.

Why is this such a resonant joke?

Because it's quick and dark and hits you before you see it coming.

Another guy walks into a doctor's office—

\* \* \*

"How are you?" Dr. Moscowitz asks. He seems genuinely interested. A kind man with a full head of white hair and a smooth, roseate complexion he has been my doctor for a decade. We're in his office at the NYU Medical Center on a warm afternoon in late May. Bill Clinton is president, Nirvana the biggest band in America. Czechoslovakia has just ceased its existence and I would much rather be in Prague drinking pilsner alongside the celebrating citizens of the spanking new Czech Republic toasting their playwright president Vaclav Havel than getting poked and prodded in the doctor's office. It is 1993 and I am thirty-seven.

To the doctor's question I respond that I am fine, as if there could be any other answer. How else should I be? My last medical drama was a college case of mononucleosis. Three weeks in bed with stabbing throat pain but in the end, cured. Since then, nothing. I play basketball and work out regularly, don't smoke, drink moderately, and am monogamous so no pesky microbes lurking in my system waiting to flower into something hard to explain. Sitting on Dr. Moscowitz's examination table in my briefs, I am a picture of apple-cheeked vigor, blazing with life.

The room is bright, cheerful. This exam an item on a to-do list, something to take care of between dropping off the dry-cleaning and picking up our takeout dinner at Chirpin' Chicken. It is with some surprise that I notice Dr. Moscowitz spending an inordinate amount of time kneading the sides of my neck. What could be on the sides of my neck? Anatomy was never my subject and I have always thought the neck was there to sheathe the throat and some bones that, if broken, would cause extraordinary problems. My throat feels fine and my bones are intact. What is he looking for? Before I can ask him, he moves his probing hands south where he finds something unusual below deck. Swollen lymph glands, he reports, in your neck and your groin, something an antibiotic should eliminate. Well, that's good enough for me. Who doesn't love an antibiotic? And what are lymph glands, anyway? Get dressed and forget about it.

\* \* \*

I am writing these words in my Los Angeles home office overlooking the Santa Monica Mountains more than two decades after that encounter with Dr. Moscowitz. Bookshelves painted white and crammed to capacity line three of the pale yellow walls. Hardbacks, paperbacks, various editions of my novels, and an arm's-length of handwritten journals that I've been keeping for over forty years. The shelves are festooned with knickknacks like a bobblehead doll of the basketball player Jamal Crawford, a ceramic cup made by my daughter, pictures of family. On one wall is a charcoal drawing of my mother. On another artfully framed snapshots of a considerably younger me leaping off a pile of rocks in what was then called Burma. My writing desk is made of pine and on it rest several books, a Peter Max ashtray, three pieces of stamped bronze metal art the size of silver dollars given to me by the Israeli artist Menashe Kadishman. I sit in an ergonomic black leather chair, worn and ripped. The carpet is a functional blue that would not be out of place on a Delta flight from Los Angeles to New York. A laptop computer is open to a Word document.

This morning before arriving at my desk I went for a four-mile hike. Despite a few age-related dings, I am in rude health. For years I have been struggling to write about what happened in the wake of that doctor visit. I've perused my journals, interrogated the people who were there. It was a year of great agitation. Fitting the memories into a coherent pattern is a way for me to better comprehend how I came to arrive where I am now. People close to me have died. I'm no longer young and don't know what I'll be able to recall in the future so I'm trying to understand how I changed as a result of what occurred before the ability to do so slips away. Before I slip away.

When my brother and I toast, we say: to the ancestors.

Arriving at a doctor's office for the first time, a nurse will hand you a clipboard with a form on it. The heading on the form reads FAMILY HISTORY. If those words had musical accompaniment, it would be comprised of sinister minor chords played on a large pipe organ, the sounds of which linger in the air long after the organist has lifted her fingers from the keys, leaving your cell structure vibrating like a tuning fork. Some families are cancer families, others heart disease. They're usually one or the other. Mine, unfortunately, is both. If there is a third disease half the world dies from, we would probably have that in our genes, too.

When it comes to family health, no one's forebears are innocent. All suffer from the original sin of decay. On this clipboard the patient is meant to list the various maladies that felled their dynasty. Aunt Iris had gout, Grandpa Lou suffered from colitis, that please-don't-tell-me-about-it-at-a-dinner-party kind of detail. The thinking goes like this: if there is a history of certain ailments it will behoove us to pay more attention to their possible presence in this individual whom we are now examining since these maladies might be *hereditary*.

I always assumed I came from healthy stock until I realized I believed that because I'd never actually thought about it. Like many humans, I am adept at not thinking about bad things. This is called *avoidance* and it is the evolutionary development that allows us to get out of bed in the morning. While I blithely trusted my family tree was bursting with green leaves, each pulsing in photosynthetic dialogue with its lustrous branch-mates, the wood was infested with termites, and about to disintegrate.

At an engagement party being held for my parents in the 1950s, one of my mother's uncles approached my father and announced, Welcome to the family. We're bleeders. Dad was appalled, but not deterred, and he married my mother as scheduled, despite this waving of the bloody red flag.

I have often taken my cues from my father. We look alike—tall, slender, beak-nosed—and our personalities share certain similarities as well. He was an "A" type who eventually learned, under my mother's patient yet unremitting tutelage, to camouflage his battering ram tendencies with copious filigrees of charm. Always nattily turned out, for years he affected colorful bowties and suspenders as visual signifiers reflecting his aversion to going along with the sartorial throng. There was no one who embodied the razzamatazz of Madison Avenue more than Leo Greenland, who was once the subject of a full-page photograph in the *New York Times* where he appeared seated at a sidewalk table with a bar code stenciled on his forehead. He loved the life, pitching new business, creating national ad campaigns, winning Clio Awards. Mondays, he once told me, could never arrive soon enough. And yet at the risk of veering, or rather crashing headfirst, into sentimentality, nothing was more important to him than my mother, my brother, and me. By any reasonable definition a positive role model, unlike my paternal grandfather, who was, to be generous, a rapscallion. To be less generous, well—why be less generous? He's my grandfather. A Polish immigrant of the non-Slavic variety, married four times before it was socially acceptable, he never earned the love of his second son, my father. When Dad was five years old, my grandfather attempted to teach him to swim at Coney Island by throwing him into the surf where he nearly drowned. Their relationship went downhill from there.

By the early 1960s, to escape his creditors, my grandfather

had moved to Los Angeles. While there he accidentally drove over the side of Coldwater Canyon with his fourth wife. Let me put this in context: Coldwater Canyon is a high, winding road with a mountain on one side and a precipitous drop on the other. To breach the railing in your car is, ordinarily, to die. But this particular bit of bad driving miraculously did not kill him (or her). He emerged from the accident with a leg brace and lived another couple of years before dying from heart problems. I met him once when I was eight years old. He took us to eat at Lawry's, a restaurant on La Cienega Boulevard famous for prime rib. I sat on his knee and remember the strange sensation of his leg brace beneath me, like a human jungle gym. When my grandfather died in 1964, Dad did not attend the funeral. At the time the profundity of this absence eluded me. Years later, my father and I drove to Forest Lawn Cemetery to search for my grandfather's grave. It was a smoggy afternoon and we had come to the San Fernando Valley from the other side of the hills. Forest Lawn is epic, an endless landscape of markers that call to mind the rolling graveyard fields in Flanders. Under a bleached southern California sun, we looked this way and that, holding a map we had been given in the office. After a twenty-minute search, there was my progenitor's stone. It read *Beloved Husband*. Those were the only words. You will recall from the prologue that the man had three children. Dad absorbed the visual, exhaled through his nose, and uttered this immortal comment: "Even in death, he *zetzes* me." For non-Yiddish speakers, "zetz" is a verb, the loose definition of which is to poke with a sharp stick.

The best thing I can say about my paternal grandfather is he didn't have cancer.

My father used my grandfather as a template of what *not* to be as a parent. And he succeeded to the degree that Dad became a model for me of what *to* be. Involved where my grandfather was uninvolved, caring where he was uncaring, and most important, *there* when my grandfather was not there.

And my father was always healthy! I use the exclamation point purposefully because Dad's nearly lifelong health is important in the context of this story. I don't remember him ever missing a day at the office until he retired at seventy-five. From him I inherited male pattern baldness and the eyesight of a cave fish. Neither are life-threatening. In my early adulthood, I was hoping to tread the same physical path as he into a vigorous old age. Then a fly landed in the proverbial ointment when he was sixty bringing with it a diagnosis of lymphoma. However, and this is a big however, it was a very mild form where a cancerous lymph node was removed and he had to take a pill for a while.

That was it.

A pill.

A big cancer scare that amounted to the smallest of potatoes. His last pill ingested, Dad continued along as if nothing had happened. Heart ailments took both my paternal grandparents in their early seventies, so this cancer lightning bolt came from a distinctly different zip code. His heart was fine. Then his older brother died of brain cancer. The noose around my neck constricted. But my uncle, a low-key furniture salesman who had followed my grandfather from New York to California, did not resemble Dad physically or in personality. They were siblings you could not quite believe were related. I was clinging to the notion that whatever hereditary mischief might be afoot would come exclusively from my father.

My mother's side of the family was more complicated. My maternal grandfather smoked, drank, ate horribly—the hacky joke here would be something along the lines of *his blood type was pastrami*—and never had cancer. Of course, he suffered eleven heart attacks, and here I will point out that the number eleven is not being invoked as comic hyperbole, before this mighty Hebraic rock, a man who had kept his extended family employed in the newspaper distribution business during the depths of the Depression, someone who had managed to avoid being whacked by the mob for gambling debts, a man that spent decades married to my grandmother who was not an easy woman, was felled by a myocardial infarction at the age of seventy-three. My maternal grandmother, who had the personality of a cardiac patient but the heart of a stallion, succumbed to breast cancer after my grandfather died. My noose tightened a little more. But I didn't have breasts so I wasn't too worried. Then my mother was diagnosed with breast cancer at fifty-seven. This was a bad development for many reasons, but in the context of what I'm writing about now, it brought up *hereditary* yet again. More noose tightening. Not to the point where I was choking, but the rope around my neck was a little snug. Both my parents had been stricken. My brother is younger than I so, clearly, at least to my way of thinking, in the game of chance that is life I was next.

But I wasn't.

While staying with friends in Montauk shortly after my mother's diagnosis, I received a phone call from my parents informing me that our fourteen-year-old Irish Setter had cancer and would have to be euthanized. The *dog* had cancer! That was a bit much, although it certainly proved he was a member of the family. When he was being taken on the last walk, my parents' housekeeper, who had known him since he was a puppy, said, "Goodbye, old friend. You've had a better life than a lot of people." She was right, although it didn't make the long ride to the veterinarian any easier for my parents.

It occurs to me that ruminating on the subject of familial medical history was my way of lending some rationality to a situation that seemed as random as being struck by a falling piece of masonry. Was I not my own master, capable of free will, a solo navigator?

Apparently not.

Rather, I was one point in a constellation of compromised relatives and ancestors whose flawed DNA I shared and, whatever mask I might slip behind, unable to hide my identity from the all-seeing eye of the universe.

And who was the I to whom this was happening, the "I" previously unrevealed? The reader knows the facts, the circumstances, the time and place, but what of the interior? In 1993 I was intent on Hollywood success. Quite intent. A careerist, but an inept one. Had I been an adept careerist, I would have been living in Los Angeles where Hollywood is actually located. Instead, after a two-year foray there a decade earlier, during which I was employed writing comedy for a major television network, I had fled to Manhattan. Despite my distance from Wilshire Boulevard, I managed to book enough screenwriting work while living in New York to suggest that avoiding law school was the right move. This was important for two reasons, the first being that it allowed me to contribute to the support of a family. The second, and perhaps more psychologically essential: it impressed my father who, to his eternal credit, never discouraged me from wanting to be a writer. And it wasn't just the jobs that impressed him, but the money they represented. A child of poverty, *that* is what really concerned him. Whenever I got work, the first person I told after my wife was my father. Mindful of his abandoned literary dreams, and grateful for the launching pad his striving had provided for mine, this felt entirely natural. But it wasn't as if I was doing it for *us*, this writing business. Dad was already flourishing, not only secure in his identity but luxuriating in it. I was doing it for me. And as the oldest son, I needed his acknowledgment. My brother is more reserved than I and opted out of this familial drama early. If he wanted to impress our father, moving into an ashram and living there for four years was not the way to do it. But I was a slave to the dynamic.

We'll get back to my brother and the ashram.

Writing is the one skill where I've ever been above average and being a successful writer had become a significant part of what I viewed as my distinctiveness. There was a bohemian facet to this life choice, a thumbing of the nose at convention and authority. To be paid to conjure words, to entertain, was barely imaginable for a product of the suburbs where creativity meant working on the literary magazine and then becoming a successful patent attorney.

What did it mean to be a successful writer? Successful in my family of origin was simply defined as making a living. But I never saw it that way. A bursting bank account was fine, but I sought *artistic* achievement, and recognition for that achievement. I attended film school with several artists of great talent who by the time I had been knocking around the business for a few years had already carved out places in a firmament upon which I could only gaze enviously since things had not broken that way for me. My own Fellini-fueled dreams were derailed in Hollywood where I was a journeyman, albeit one that kept getting jobs, which beat digging ditches. And I naively kept angling for creative fulfillment, writing spec screenplays that were not the usual studio fare, pitching television shows meant to break one mold or another. This is what I was doing a few years after the Berlin Wall came down. Making a living without having achieved anything close to what I viewed as success, and early death threatened to put a crimp in these plans.

Wait, early *death*? Why was I thinking about death? Wasn't this an ordinary doctor visit? It appeared that way at first. But then the doctor found *nodes* and ordered *tests*. My mind has always run probabilities like a Las Vegas oddsmaker and variations on the catastrophic quickly come into focus. A ghastly outcome may have been unlikely, but was it possible? Of course it was. Live long enough and you know that a ghastly outcome is always possible. I tried to repress this thought but it began to buck and quickly broke free. The most challenging way to not think about death is to try and force yourself to not think about it. Was I actually going to die from whatever these nodes foretold? And if I was, how wedded was I back then to a materialistic view of the universe? Did life really just *end*?

One night in my late twenties, I found myself stone cold sober and halfway up the Great Pyramid of Cheops at Giza paralyzed by an attack of acrophobia. Along with being embarrassing, this was highly illegal. How did I come to be in this treacherous position? It was the early 80s and having finished a season on the writing staff of a television show that had me questioning my career, I wanted to get as far away from my life choices as possible. A British friend was planning a rolling house party in Egypt, did I want to join? How do you say yes in Arabic? Now I was hanging off a pyramid—we had paid a guide to take us up and the others were scampering like rabbits toward the summit. It was meant to be a lark, the kind of wild thing you do at that age, and rather than dancing a little jig at the top I had to crabwalk down on my backside as the guide slapped each successive descending stone with his palm to indicate precisely where I should place my bottom. While falling from a pyramid does not look physically possible from the photographs of the pyramids with which we're all familiar, a Dutch tourist had recently attempted the ascent and plummeted to his death. So, my adventure on the tomb of Cheops was marked largely by my own fear and disgrace, and the complex cosmology of the Egyptian afterlife represented by the stones I was slinking down escaped me entirely. And why should I have been thinking about what happens when we die? I was a young man with screenplays to write, a lifetime of experience to cultivate.

How exactly did the Egyptians view the afterlife?

Upon dying ancient Egyptians were immediately faced with Osiris, the god of the underworld, and surrounded by forty-two additional gods including the Swallower of shades, the Bone-breaker, and the Eater of entrails (If I'd been visualizing this while dangling from the pyramid, it might have made me anxious enough to fall off.) Already scared out of her wits, the newly dead Egyptian is confronted by the god Thoth in the form of a baboon, seated on a pair of scales that will decide the fate of the shaking wraith in front of him. Should the petitioner suffer a negative result a horrible second death awaits. A *second* death! Because one was not enough. It should be a relief to learn that the person undergoing this trial is armed with the Book of the Dead in which tips for surviving the hereafter are helpfully dispensed. They have to fend off snakes, crocodiles, and insects which make the ancient Egyptian afterlife sound a lot like a Japanese game show. A journey ensues—it's not enough that your life has ended, now you have to go on a trip—but there are many versions of the Egyptian Book of the Dead, so there is no conclusive end point. You could wind up sailing blissfully with the sun god Ra for all eternity, or in the Field of Reeds, where the departed endlessly pursue an idealized simulacrum of their earthly lives with good food, drink, and lots of sex, which makes the Field of Reeds a progenitor of both the Christian idea of Heaven and the all-inclusive Caribbean resort.

Are their notions any more absurd than ours?

I mention all of this to suggest the mind-numbing detail with which this question has been chewed over since the development of language. The riddle of what happens when we die is no closer to being settled than the one that asks whether LeBron James is better at basketball than Michael Jordan. Although there is no written record of the thoughts and preoccupations of Early Man, one can guess that as soon as the ability to think abstractly evolved, serious thought was given to the matter of non-being. Let me take you back to the Pleistocene Era—one day, your neighbor is happily existing in his cave, the next he is dead. He was there and then his body is there but he, apparently, is not. Limbs lifeless, eyes dull, once warm body now cold. What happened? Who can explain such a thing? The forebears of future New Yorkers ask: Is his cave now available? Religion evolved to help resolve this matter and the writers of the texts of the world's major faiths gave a great deal of attention to this component of their respective dogmas.

I wish I could tell you that today I barely consider the subject at all, yet this would not be true. I think about it often. But the California sky is a dome of brilliant blue, the temperature is in the eighties, and when I'm done working this afternoon I'll go to the movies.

How often do *you* think about dying?

\* \* \*

Still reeling from my troubling audience with Dr. Moscowitz, I emerge from the subway at 72nd Street and cross Broadway toward Amsterdam Avenue. Gray's Papaya is filled with the usual herd of discriminating gourmands wolfing cheap hot dogs chased with the eponymous orangey drink. New York street food is in my blood and it's tempting to get a fix, but I head north. The Upper West Side of Manhattan is my home. Where I live and work.

It was July four years earlier when Susan and I moved in together. I had been existing in a studio on West 57th and she was in a small, ground floor one bedroom on West 74th Street that had been a dentist's office. Being wily, Susan was able to persuade her landlord to rent us a much larger two-bedroom in a building he owned on West 76th Street at what was considered a reasonable rate. The building was hardly fancy and the middle-aged doorman whose name was Vito displayed a predilection for Nazi-related literature; other than that, we were thrilled.

But: It was adjacent to Riverside Memorial Chapel.

Since our new home was to be on the third floor, we would be sharing a living room wall with a building full of corpses. I tried not to think about it but couldn't stop. How was I supposed to exist in my new home, splayed on the sofa reading a novel or listening to music or just watching the traffic float up Amsterdam Avenue, knowing that in the immediate vicinity was a never-ending parade of dead people. New ones constantly arriving to replace the ones being carted away. There is a morbid streak in me, but it does not go this far. I discussed it with Susan, who did not have any problem being neighbors with the newly deceased. After further rumination, the following conclusion was reached: with a two-bedroom apartment in the west 70s, unless the corpses rose zombified from the dead and began to eat flesh, I would keep my feelings to myself.

On the day we moved in, predictably, there was a funeral taking place. It was bad enough knowing that what lay on the other side of the wall was a carnival of death. Every day a sidewalk choked with mourners. A steady diet of dead people and those who love them milling around discussing the *death* of the *deceased*. Who were incontrovertibly *dead*. A perpetual *Diá de los Muertos*.

This was our new life.

But it was not just any funeral on that hot summer day. They were saying *kaddish* for Steve Rubell, the co-owner of Studio 54, a nightclub in New York that for a period in the late 1970s was the epicenter of disco decadence, a Caligulan environment of powdery drugs, polymorphous sex, and catchy bad music.

Oh, Disco Apollo, how brightly you shined! Because of a mass desire on the part of the hoi polloi to see and be seen with the celebrities of the day, no one who was not rich or beautiful could get into this club. It was the beginning of today's velvet rope culture; a place defined by its exclusivity, its ability to make average people feel even more average. Desperate lines snaked down 54th Street and around the corner, bridge and tunnel types mixing with urbanites, hipsters, fashionistas, Wall Streeters, gays and straights, huddled masses yearning to breathe the carcinogenic air inside. Burly bouncers would point—*You, in. You, go back to Queens.* The rejected would skulk down the sidewalk wondering how their lives could have gone so wrong, while the elect would assume their rightful places among the pantheon of the previously anointed.

It was the kind of club where a large glittery moon would periodically descend from the ceiling to be met by a long, equally glittery spoon. The spoon zeroed in on the moon's nose, then—snort! And the pulsating, sweaty crowd would celebrate anew. At the time, people considered this cocaine sight gag to be the height of cultural mischief. It was the decade in a shiny nutshell—sparkling and dumb. The boldface names of the era were there every night, dancing and drugging, enveloped in the drum and bass throb, the flashing lights, the sensory overload. Steve Rubell presided over this night world of eternal youth; its Mordred, its dark prince. But punk vaporized disco, then Steve Rubell got AIDS and died at forty-five. This diminutive disco supernova who had towered above the Manhattan demimonde like a cocaine-fueled colossus, was already forgotten. Oh, sure, the odd window dresser, fashion designer, or Liza buff remembered him, but his days as a household name were over. He was ancient history, as relevant as Toots Shor or Texas Guinan, noteworthy saloonistas of their own day, now unrecalled.

*Alas, poor Steve, I knew him . . .*

His death would not have reverberated were they not having his funeral next door to the new apartment. I am generally not a person who thinks about omens. Things go wrong naturally enough without worrying about omens. That said—this was not a good one.

And yet.

After a few weeks, no one thinks about neighbors unless they're fighting. The revolving dead became part of the psychic wallpaper. There was a florist on the block, and a Burmese restaurant, and then there was Riverside Memorial Chapel. Just businesses. People making a living. Flowers, noodles, and death—they all ran together in the wash of life. Even the throngs of mourners gathered on the sidewalk several times a week ceased to register.

Now as I walk past the Burmese restaurant on the way home from Dr. Moscowitz's office, all is well. As I walk past the flower shop, all is well. But as I walk past Riverside the carapace I have constructed cracks for a moment and I glance over and see Death leering through the wide front doors of this memorial palace, this house of farewell, winking, beckoning passersby to the chapel, the casket, the corpse. Doesn't everyone sense this mordant presence, or is it only me? I shudder. Instead of walking directly home, I get the antibiotic prescription filled at a drugstore on Broadway. I can't get better fast enough. This pharmacy is where we buy toothpaste, deodorant, and soap, commonplace things for routine days. We have had prescriptions filled here any number of times. We always take the medicine and it always works because that's what medicine does in our predictable world. I assure myself there is nothing different today. Dr. Moscowitz has examined me annually for the past seven years. There is never anything wrong.

\* \* \*

When I described my California office a few pages back, there was one photograph I didn't mention. An image of Susan and me paddling an inflatable rubber raft. Are we shooting the rapids in a flume of Idaho whitewater risking life and limb? Navigating the tranquil shore of tree-lined Lake Superior, two intrepid voyagers silhouetted against the vast northern Michigan sky? No, we're in a beat-up swimming pool in the backyard of a rambling old house in a Hudson River town. The effect is mildly comical and the photograph a helpful reminder not to ever take ourselves too seriously. It is that sensibility we share, one that acknowledges the difficulty of maintaining an old-school sense of dignity while navigating the capricious tides of human existence, that made me fall in love with the woman in the raft.

On a humid August afternoon some years earlier there was a party at a friend's suburban New York backyard. Accompanying me was my girlfriend with whom I had been living for nearly four years in a SoHo walk-up with a shower in the kitchen and water bugs the size of hamsters. It was an artist's garret, and I was there to do what artists do: pay as little rent as possible while trying to figure out how to monetize my single skill.

Another woman was at the party with her considerably older fiancé. They lived downtown too, not far from us, but I had never seen her before. Blonde hair chopped short, plaid miniskirt with a black top, and Doc Martens. A wry smile, an acerbic sense of humor. Instantly, I was smitten. When I found out she worked for Orion Pictures, a company that made actual movies, the kind people paid to see in theaters, I was in her thrall. My days were being spent as an associate producer of a television show called *Good Morning, New York*, a program constructed from equal parts inane chat and celebrity self-promotion—Arnold Schwarzenegger, James Mason, Matt Dillon, Senator John Glenn, Joe Namath, Richard Simmons, and Divine were denizens of our green room—but television was a detour. I hadn't gone to film school so I could write intros to be chirped by the twinkly hostess of a breakfast show, *ladies and gentlemen, please welcome Dr. Ruth Westheimer.* I would be a screenwriter. This sylph-like blonde with the short skirt and the fiancé who looked two weeks away from a hip replacement had managed to break into the movie business, no small feat in New York City. We chattered as we ate our hamburgers; I flirted madly. A week later I took a trip to Los Angeles. I remained there for the next two years. My girlfriend and I broke up. People have asked me whether I ever did stand-up comedy. It is with a certain degree of regret that I tell them that when it came to telling jokes into a microphone to a room of drunken strangers my courage was not that of a thousand lions. But it was during an early Reagan-era winter that I seriously considered it. I hung out at the Comedy Store on Sunset Boulevard most nights. One comic was a misogynistic former preacher who wore a long wool coat and screeched at the audience. He killed. There was an act who pulled a surgical glove over his head and blew it up so he looked like a cartoon rooster. He also killed. But those guys were in another lane. My strength would be the writing. I began to create an act. Several pages of a yellow legal pad scrawled with material. I worked it into a tight five minutes suitable for an open mic audition. But something essential was missing—there was no point of view. I had no "voice." Just another white guy with jokes and that was not going to cut it.

However—at that time "just another white guy with jokes" described pretty much every writer on a network sitcom and I was "staffed," a verb that does not exist east of Los Angeles and means hired as a staff writer. When you are a young writer and have not yet developed a voice this is an excellent gig since it consists of putting words in the mouths of pre-existing characters, thereby short-circuiting the heavy lifting of actual creativity. In the early 1980s "quality" television was experiencing a revival. Unfortunately, the show that hired me was not part of the trend but given that the previous several months had been spent selling cable television subscriptions door to door in the barrio—you have not lived until you have tried to convince a Mexican immigrant who does not speak English and probably thinks you're from the Immigration and Naturalization Service and are about to deport him that he should purchase HBO and Showtime—it represented a significant step up.

A septuagenarian John Houseman, of whom I was in such awe that whenever I mustered the courage to talk to him I stuttered, was a cast member of the first show I worked on. He had co-founded the Mercury Theatre with Orson Welles in the 1930s and he could have had no illusions about the value of what we were doing since he was concurrently appearing in Volvo commercials. But his mere presence provided an education in the *realpolitik* of the entertainment business—work when you can. The paycheck was, for someone who had been showering in a tenement walk-up, two feet from where he ate cornflakes, mind-boggling, and its weekly arrival made me an official Hollywood writer.

But the job was not without stress.

Unless you have been a defendant in a criminal trial, nothing prepares you for the pressure of being fresh meat in the Writers Room. Sitcoms are put together on the industrial model, and the conveyor belt starts with the script. The factory hands (i.e. writers) sit around a table picking at bad food and moaning about their over-privileged lives while banging out stories and jokes. Jokes were money. The room was often entirely male and, as with all high testosterone environments, nurturing as a firing squad. Because you were being judged every time you opened your mouth, the pressure to be laugh out loud funny—smiles and sardonic grins were poor substitutes—particularly for a newcomer, was intense. Everyone there had a friend who needed a job and was funnier than you; what the hell were you doing there anyway? Silence was not an option. Silence was an admission that you couldn't be funny in the room, doom for a comedy writer. So, like a hungry bear standing by a salmon stream, you waited for an opportunity, and waited, and then—you pounced. If you scored, and cracked everyone up, the dopamine burst was blinding. There was nothing quite like getting a roomful of jaded comedy writers to stop complaining long enough to laugh at something you said. For that moment, you were the most popular, successful, best-looking guy in the room. You owned it. But if you bombed, it was death. The stillness of the crypt. The upside: the ignominy was brief, others would eventually resume pitching, and someone else was bound to bomb soon so your colleagues would forget how incompetent you were. Then you'd score, laughter would reign, liberally seasoned with the envy of everyone who hadn't said what caused it, and all would be forgotten.

Pitching story ideas was less of a high-wire act since whatever anyone suggested, no matter how lame, would often lead to something more fruitful. Another writer might pick up your idea, modify it slightly, sprinkle some fairy dust, and then the whole room was off to the races.

You could even preface your remarks by saying Here's the bad version. The bad version was a placeholder intended to move the narrative forward until a more elegant solution could be found. Occasionally, someone would hear a bad version and say something like, Wait, that might work. But not often.

"Let's give the character a problem."

"What's the bad version?"

"He has cancer."

Occasionally, you would be sent off to work on a script. The story had already been vetted in the room, so this consisted of writing the actual dialogue for all the scenes and making everything flow. When this process was complete, the script, your precious baby, was served to the writers' room, where it was worked over like a mob informant who has fallen into the hands of those he has betrayed. By the time it had been "fixed," it was virtually unrecognizable. There is a famous anecdote concerning the playwright George S. Kaufman, who was hired to write a show for the Marx Brothers. While seated in the back of the theater at a preview, he is reported to have said, "Shhh! I think I just heard one of my lines." This is the lot of the comedy writer.

I moved to another show to work with a famous producer. A rising Latino comedian was going to play a fictional version of himself. The show would be groundbreaking, the first sitcom about Latinos. Television history would be made. Everyone anticipated a long run.

The project did not set the world on its ear. I sensed the show might be slightly off-key when the fictional comic's Mexican-American nieces and nephews made their first entrance in the pilot episode; so many kids ran through the door it looked like a fire drill at a daycare center.

Apparently, America did not want to see this because the series had a toe tag after six episodes. A show that was going to be shot in New York hired me and I traveled back there for six weeks. By the end of the first day—over a beer with a friend at Jimmy Day's on Sheridan Square, a place where the sidewalks were filled with actual people—I knew that when I flew west it would be to pack up my apartment.

But there was another reason I broke up with Los Angeles. The single life was losing its charms and this was brought home in one particularly clarifying moment. When I moved there my only acquaintance was a louche screenwriter I barely knew, to whom I had been introduced by a mutual friend. Let's call him Dennis. To my relief, he took me under his disreputable wing, let me crash at his place, and shared secret knowledge of the movie business (he knew nothing, I later learned). We became friends with a waitress named

Charlene and one night the three of us found ourselves drunk, stoned, and naked in a hot tub. As one did in 1982 in Los Angeles where most conversations to which I was privy were either about Hollywood or the prospect of nuclear annihilation. While I was ruminating on Ronald Reagan's relationship with the Soviet leader Yuri Andropov, or Nietzsche's law of eternal return, or anything to keep from wondering how I came to find myself drunk, stoned, and naked in hot tub with two near-strangers, Dennis and Charlene began to nuzzle which was clearly a prelude to what was going to be aquatic sex and with a subtle gesture in my direction, Dennis indicated that the three of us should start collaborating. Here was my opportunity! The chance to be a young, footloose screenwriting sybarite, drinking and drugging and fucking his way through Los Angeles and right in front of me was the sex-all-the-time legacy of previous decades being served on a watery platter. But I never felt more desolate than I did at that moment in that hot tub, more alienated, more ridiculous. Three-ways are better left to those more willing to share and I retreated to the confines of a nearby sauna consumed by existential discontents while Dennis and Charlene capered in the churning water like a pair of amphibious rabbits.

Los Angeles, I thought, you are not for me.

In all this time, I continued to think about my witty film business crush with the plaid skirt, black pullover, and Doc Martens. Two years expired. I called my friend at whose backyard party we had briefly mingled. It was five years later.

"What happened to that girl I met at your house, the cute one in the plaid skirt?"

"She just got divorced."

My timing was that of a trapeze artist. Never was anyone's marital woe more welcome news. My friend gave me her phone number and I called. We made a date for a few days hence. I could barely contain myself. On the day of the date, she tried to beg off because she was sick. She actually *was* sick but I had been waiting five years and did not want to wait another day. I cajoled and inveigled. There was some token resistance but I eventually persuaded her. We attended a book party and had dinner at an Italian restaurant on Amsterdam Avenue. I was so enamored from the moment I picked her up that my adrenaline kicked into overdrive and I found myself narrating much of our evening as it went along. It was not an internal monologue. Susan heard every word. The memory makes me wince.

"I think we're having a good time, aren't we?"

"Umm—"

"You seem to be enjoying yourself."

"Well—"

She survived my performance and as we were saying goodnight amazingly agreed a second date which she did not try to cancel. Three years later we got married. I was ambivalent about the idea of getting married and proposed three times. She said yes each time, but somehow I contrived to retract each offer. The first time I asked her not to tell anyone that I had proposed. Then I hoped she would forget that it had happened. The second time I proposed and immediately developed a significant if temporary problem with my digestive tract and although I am not proud of typing the words "explosive diarrhea," scrupulous honesty compels me to do exactly that. The problem cleared up after several days. The third time everything proceeded normally and we were married on September 8th, 1990.

It's strange to recollect the multiple proposals and how unhinged I was by the whole idea because after dating for six months, I knew I wanted to spend the rest of my life with her.

Here is how: we were traveling in Thailand and decided to take a side trip to Burma. It was in the early days of the military dictatorship and the country was tightly controlled. Tourists had to be under government supervision at all times.

Despite this, a black-market travel industry thrived. Drivers were paid in American dollars, which were closely regulated, and they guided you surreptitiously around the country, showed you this shrine, that temple, and by serving as the local Michelin Guide, kept you from bringing a case of dysentery home with your faux jade elephant. We had heard about this in Bangkok and smuggled currency into Burma in the form of three hundred single American dollars stuffed into my undershorts.

Near the veranda of our hotel in Rangoon chatting with a group of hustlers was a guide who called himself Lawrence because his Burmese name was unpronounceable to my sclerotic American tongue and he agreed to meet us the following day before dawn. The army did not put up roadblocks until after their morning tea—it was not the world's most efficient dictatorship—so there was a sizable exodus of people out of the city each day before the checkpoints were in place.

The next morning we climbed into the bed of Lawrence's pickup truck and left Rangoon for the drive north. For twelve hours, we sat on our duffel bags as the Burmese countryside sailed past. Farms and villages surrounded by rice paddies. Thin cattle and peasants, equally thin, driving them with sticks. We climbed into the mountains at twilight and huddled together against the chill. In the gathering darkness, we saw slashes of fire blazing across mountainsides in long looping arcs. The burning seemed controlled but we were not sure. On the dark road the effect was eerie, otherworldly. There were no towns for miles now. The truck bumped along. Lawrence had brought two helpers with him who did not communicate with us. No one knew where we were. We had only told our families we were going to Thailand. Lawrence informed us twelve hours earlier we were headed for an old British hill station built during the Raj. In the early morning, we had visions of lawn tennis and Pimms Cup. Now we were wondering if Lawrence and his confederates were going to kill us in the flaming mountains. Exchanging nervous glances, we rode it out. It was not as if we could walk anywhere. Then there were lights in the distance and they were not coming from a burning mountainside. It was the hill station. Exhausted and covered in grit from the ride, we checked into a hotel that resembled an English country estate. It was the farthest away from home either of us had ever been. Our second-floor room was large and airy. Through the leaded panes of an ancient window the lawn tennis court I envisioned appeared as if in a Victorian reverie. Then Susan walked into the bathroom and discovered the toilet was a hole in the floor with two rubber pads on either side to put your feet.

"Well, then," said this well-respected, fashionable lawyer on holiday from her high-stress job at a major broadcast network, "do you think this place has a bar?"

At that moment, it became clear who I wanted to push my wheelchair.

\* \* \*

With the antibiotic in my pocket, the elixir, the answer to what I keep trying to assure myself is my perfectly ordinary problem, I arrive home from the doctor's office trying without much success to banish thoughts of his fingers on my neck. In a recent and misguided attempt to escape the tyranny of white we have painted our apartment shades of burnt umber and teal, colors more at home on the ceramic plates festooning the walls of second-rate Mexican restaurants, and have recently had several conversations in which we questioned our decision as well as our general design sense. None of this is on my mind as I enter the apartment. Susan is making spaghetti for dinner. Four months pregnant, her stomach remains flat. A high-wattage lawyer who girds for work in pumps and power suits, she has doffed the Ann Taylor drag and slipped into jeans. Our almost two-year-old daughter Allegra plays on the living room floor. As Susan stirs the sauce, I consider my good fortune. My wife is lovely enough to play the lead in a television drama about young lawyers. Although physical exercise is her kryptonite, even pregnant she still has the trim figure of an athlete. Straight, silky blonde hair falls over her shoulders. Her face is open and sympathetic, the face of someone who usually gives people more time than they deserve. She asks me how my routine physical went.

I tell her it was fine.

Susan's presence is like a quilt. She grew up in a house on a lake in southwestern Michigan, the youngest daughter of a civil engineer who enjoyed a cocktail and a housewife that suffered the consequences. Her siblings are twins, a brother and sister, three years older. Summers on the Upper Peninsula, moose territory. Gray Lake Superior vistas, pristine white sand beaches, the northern water so cold the fish are shivering. Cornish pasties and Vernor's Ginger Ale. At sixteen, she drove a truck for the public works department. In college, she was a theatre major and after graduating migrated to New York to intern as an assistant in the opera department at Juilliard, although her own tastes run more to Steve Earle and Willie Nelson. Ultimately more practical than a career making magic would allow, she earned a law degree. We fit like a Fender Telecaster guitar in a plush case.

I pour myself a beer and tell Susan about my visit with Dr. Moscowitz.

She's watching her network's evening news on a small countertop television. At work, she handles sexual harassment claims. A certain mega-profile employee at the network has inspired a line to form outside her office.

"Swollen glands?" she says, looking away from a story about a political scandal in Queens.

"I'm sure it's nothing."

Susan agrees. Her demeanor implies that there will be plenty of time for hysteria should that be necessary but tonight we will eat pasta and play with our daughter. Can you feast on someone's demeanor? I feast on Susan's.

"Have you heard of Schrodinger's Cat?" I say.

"What about it?" she asks, stirring the sauce.

"Doesn't that describe how all of us are living?"

"In a closed box with a cyanide vial and radiation not knowing if we're alive or dead?" In goes more oregano. She tastes the sauce.

"Not that we don't know if we're living or dead, but whether we're closer to life or closer to death."

"You have swollen glands. You're not closer to death."

"It's an imperfect analogy but we really have no idea what's going on with us on a cellular level. No idea at all. We could be perfectly healthy or have a fatal disease and there's a chance that for a while at least we won't know which one it is."

"Why are you thinking like this?" She drains the pasta. "You're probably fine."

"I'm just trying to get comfortable with the uncertainty."

"No one is ever comfortable with uncertainty." She pauses. "Do you think you can make a salad?"

As for the red sauce and its seasoning of tarragon, basil, and oregano, I can barely taste it through the apprehension. We don't return to the problem of Schrodinger's Cat. Instead, we read to Allegra and then put her to bed. She doesn't like to be left alone and the howling begins shortly after Susan walks out of her bedroom. It is primal, unremitting, and builds in intensity. It contains untold agonies. To my empathic ears, it is like the wail of an animal caught in a trap and it echoes the sound in my head, one that Susan cannot hear, the aria of my anxiety.

Recently, Susan read a book by a widely respected sadist

called Dr. Richard Ferber and it is his advice we are following. The thinking is that if you allow the baby to sleep in your bed, an unhealthy attachment will develop. But Allegra's bellowing is a blessing this evening since it is keeping me from focusing on my visit with Dr. Moscowitz. Our daughter's crying is annoying, aggravating even, but it is also grounding.

Over the next week I attend a Knicks game, have two business lunches, see some friends, go to several movies, and take a full course of antibiotics. Another visit to Dr. Moscowitz. Again, he kneads my neck like pizza dough, feels around my groin. A look of concern blossoms on his face. Concern is never something you want to see blossoming on the face of your internist. Interest, certainly. Boredom, even. But concern? Never. Concern is a portent, a foreshadowing. Thunder in the distance, the tinkling of wind chimes as the sky darkens.

In an unnerving development, the swelling has not responded to the drugs and further tests are ordered. My stomach drops three inches.

The radiologist who administers the sonogram, Dr. Yee, looks at the screen as he waves the wand over my abdomen like he's expecting to conjure a dove out of my navel and asks me if I've been traveling recently. I tell him no. Dr. Yee is young and has not developed the poker face necessary to his profession. Although he tells me nothing, his features momentarily shift into a look of barely concealed alarm before reverting to professional disinterest. He doesn't know that he has a tell. The thunder closer now, chased by flashes of lightning.

That evening my father calls and I tell him what's going on, trying to keep the apprehension out of my voice. Susan insists we consult with Dr. Moscowitz as soon as possible. Sleep is elusive that night and the next morning she and I are camped in his waiting room. New York doctors' offices are run with the protocol of a NASA launch, and what you don't do is turn up without an appointment. Susan is unbothered by this and I am too anxious to care. The nurses, versed in the ways of hysteria, take our presence in stride.

We wait. Then we wait some more. Dr. Moscowitz makes us wait all morning. Finally, just before the lunch hour, we are admitted to the inner sanctum. My nerves crackle. Palms sweating, I wipe them on my knees. Dr. Moscowitz asks me to take an AIDS test and have a CAT scan of my groin, abdomen, and chest. Groin, abdomen, *and* chest? That can't be good. Sensing my anxiety, likely visible from an aerial photograph, he arranges for the tests to take place that afternoon.

For the scan, I drink four glasses of viscous barium that tastes like liquid chalk. They park me on a gurney, jam a needle in my arm, and slide me into a big electronic donut where three-dimensional photographs are taken of my quaking guts. I stare at the ceiling and try not to think about my expiration date.

Meanwhile, a biopsy is scheduled. Gone are the X-ray machines, sharpen the knives. The procedure is to be performed by the head of surgery the following Wednesday, nearly a week away. More waiting? A week's worth, when who knows what is germinating below the surface, mutating, preparing to burst forth and wreak havoc? Susan explains to my doctor this is not acceptable. She informs him we don't need the head of surgery—anyone who knows how to extract a lymph gland will be fine, the Korean guy who slices lox at Zabar's will do in a pinch. Miraculously, she arranges for an appointment with a surgeon the following day. Susan is one of those people who can be overwhelmed by the mundane, but when it comes to something earthshaking, there is no one better. *Negotiate a nuclear pact with Russia? No problem, if I can just find the car keys.*

A valium almost allows me to sleep that night. What if I actually have *cancer?* What if I'm going to *die?* Sure, Dad had cancer and *he* didn't die but he grew up poor, served in the Army, and became successful with no one's help. He's way tougher than I am; more of a fighter. What will happen to me? Will I, in a few short years (Months? Weeks? Days?) be lying in a hospital bed surrounded by family as my organs shut down one by one, first unable to swallow, then unable to see, hearing muted sounds in the distance until, finally, a faint murmur, someone's voice fading, fading, and then—and then? I stop thinking about *that* as the inner seas pitch and heave and my mind goes reeling in the opposite direction, farther and farther back, past marriage and early adulthood and college and high school and adolescence to my parents' first house, a split-level on a middle-class cul de sac, and one of my first conscious memories: a summer day and I am standing in the kitchen, green grass visible through the window bright in the suburban afternoon. My mother has turned on the electric stove to heat food for our lunch. I watch the coils of the burner begin to turn a shade of red I have never seen. It has oranges in it, and pinks and yellows. I'm hypnotized by this moon-shaped color-shifting heat conductor.

My mother smiles at me. She has an oval face and her auburn hair is pulled into bun. She is twenty-seven years old. On that day I am her only child. Her love is perfect. She will always protect me. She turns away for a moment and I place my soft palm flat on the electric burner.

I scream. A provocateur. An explorer.

The tired morning staggers in. *Seinfeld* was on the night before. One of the subplots involved George Costanza getting a biopsy and waiting for the results. Since it is not the kind of show where anyone gets cancer, the results were negative. I hoped that was an omen, and not of the Steve Rubell's funeral variety. It is possible to think that way because I have chosen to ignore that I'd dropped five pounds over the past month. It had not occurred to me that I might already be fading away, a dimming image, an erased cartoon.

My father gives us a ride to the hospital. I sit in the passenger seat and Susan slides in behind me. As a driver, Dad hails from the Formula One school. His philosophy, which he is happy to share, is "fill the empty spaces." The technique is a metaphor for his personality. This morning, as he zooms and darts his way downtown, the car is silent. What is there to say? That when you are simply going along and living your life, you can be struck, completely out of the blue, by a meteor?

The car slows for a red light at Columbus Circle before easing to a stop. Then, without warning, we are jolted, knocked, *slammed* forward.

Another car has crashed into us.

Because—of course.

I'm going to the hospital to find out whether despite feeling perfectly healthy I have cancer which would be like getting rear-ended by another car when we are literally rear-ended by another car.

It turns out *that* was the omen.

After determining no one has been injured, Susan and I leave Dad to deal with the person who caused the accident—I was too distracted to register their identity—and take a cab the rest of the way. We arrive without a safe falling on us from a high window.

The surgeon is a young woman named Dr. Amber Guth. She is around my age and her physical beauty is distracting. The tranquilizer she gives me comes as a great relief. Lying on the operating table, pants around my ankles, I show her where the problem is. When Dr. Guth is simply talking, her presence evokes that of a model, but once she begins to perform her surgical function she becomes one of those rare female doctors whose appearance is not so much that of a doctor but, rather, that of an actress who plays a doctor on television. This makes me think about Susan, a lawyer who looks like an actress who plays a lawyer on television. The sense of acting a scene in a medical drama overtakes me and I am momentarily disturbed by the notion that I am watching entirely too much television. I think about a movie Nicole Kidman made early in her career. She played a brain surgeon and, in a collective abdication of critical responsibility, many reviewers pointed out that there could not be any brain surgeons who looked like Nicole Kidman. My mind swings back to the doctor, at least as attractive as Nicole Kidman, and the sharp object she is wielding in this scene that we are enacting that is not a dramatic scene but my actual life. Despite my surgeon's highly alluring qualities, there is no danger of an erection at this moment due to a combination of the glinting scalpel's proximity to my genitals and the effectiveness of the tranquilizer.

A local anesthetic is administered and my starlet/surgeon goes to work, slicing me like a cantaloupe. The whole process takes forty-five minutes during which I am surprisingly relaxed. Not Miles Davis *Kind of Blue* relaxed, but there is no gibbering. Dr. Guth shows me the swollen lymph gland she removed from my groin. It is a sickly, yellowish thing the size of a large fava bean.

While recovering in her office, I am buoyed by a surprise visit from Dr. Moscowitz who tells me that while the CAT scan showed some inflamed lymph nodes, there is no activity on any of my organs. This is a tremendous relief. Also, I don't have AIDS. But it's a Friday and we won't hear anything conclusive about the biopsy until the following week. One of the things I noticed during my mother's experience of being in the medical system with a serious illness is the vast number of diagnostic procedures that take place on Friday, creating countless difficult weekends, weekends built solely around distraction.

The diversion this weekend is the NBA playoffs and the Knicks are in the Eastern Conference finals. As a lifelong fan, this is close to a perfect distraction from dark thoughts. That evening I spot Doc Rivers, their starting point guard, at Tower Records on Broadway. This is a good omen, one that blurs the memory of the car accident. The omen business is getting out of hand; every encounter, impression, bit of news, a potential sign. I have been reduced to looking for omens, something you never think about when you're not looking for them. Soon I'll be examining animal entrails for signs from the universe. It does not behoove a person to inquire *how did I arrive at this state?* The answer is at once too obvious and too depressing.

The Knicks beat the Chicago Bulls in Game One on Sunday. Valium keeps the nerves from braying like a pack of donkeys and Tylenol with codeine helps me sleep. I worry I might be turning into a drug addict but I don't care. I swing from sheer terror to thinking I can handle whatever is thrown at me with a sangfroid James Bond would envy to thinking there's nothing wrong save for some virus that is definitely not AIDS.

On Monday morning, I weigh myself at the gym—where I work out all the time because I'm as healthy as those sled dogs that compete in the Iditarod! Hook six of me up to one of those contraptions and we'll pull you for a thousand miles across the tundra!—and find out the lost weight has been regained. You can't possibly regain weight if you have cancer, right? *RIGHT?!* Yes, right, of course, right. Jesus Keeeriiist, calm down.

Susan and I walk to the Barnes and Noble on 83rd Street where I read some disturbing things in a medical text that propel me into a funk for several hours. This is a violation of a cardinal rule: avoid information without context. Had I read about pleurisy, I would have been convinced I suffered from it. Perimenopause: ditto.

No word from any of the doctors yet. Someone in Dr. Guth's office tells us we probably won't get the biopsy results until Thursday.

Thursday? More waiting? How am I supposed to wait until Thursday?

Concentration is impossible. There's a new script to write, another on the horizon. It's the professional opportunity I've been auditioning for since getting out of film school. That I would be having a health crisis now is unimaginable. I can't wait for the diagnosis and the attendant dread is crippling.

*Dread*: a word I'd associated with reggae, white sand beaches, rum, poverty, jerk chicken, Red Stripe beer, and all things Jamaican since it was inevitably followed by the word *locks*. Now it is my constant companion, my Siamese twin, and I try to ignore the dread, but it tugs and pulls and nudges and doesn't want me to forget it's there.

It cannot possibly be my time.

Everything is fine.

\* \* \*

Two months after Allegra was born, twenty-seven years ago, my mother died. A little over a year before the story I'm telling you took place she was admitted to the same hospital where my lymph was removed. Susan and I brought Allegra down to visit. My mother brightened the minute her granddaughter appeared. Once, they locked eyes for nearly ten minutes, Allegra speaking her own language, cooing, gurgling noises, as my mother dandled her.

The hospital room was on the tenth floor overlooking a heliport on the East River. Each day the helicopters would come and go, people arriving, people departing. One would come in and another would take off, climbing above the river and banking into the blue distance.

My mother's illness had proceeded along a route familiar to legions of people whose lives have been invaded by cancer and its attendant miseries. Chemotherapy, tumor shrinkage, hope, recurrence, more chemotherapy, some shrinkage but not as much this time, recurrence, more hope, and disappointment.

My mother had gone into the hospital that last time expecting to be discharged. We were all expecting it since her four years of being a cancer patient had involved several hospitalizations, all of which had ended with her going home, vowing to fight on, bear up, do whatever it took for more life. And we were in denial because the sallow complexion, the hollowed cheeks that reflected the cells' inability to absorb nutrition and were diminishing her by the day, told us all we needed to know if we cared to which we did not. But the doctors made us snap out of it because they told us that this time was different, this time she would not be going home. We didn't believe them at first, having become inured to the whole idea of prognosis, something easy to do when you're watching someone you love in a mortal struggle and delusions are not easy to discard. But as her body began to shut down, subtle signs of dementia appeared indicating the cancer had metastasized to her brain, and reality intruded.

My mother decided she wanted to talk to each one of us individually, us being me, my brother, and our cousins Miles and Cori, her late, older sister's children, to whom she had been particularly close. We were all gathered in the hallway outside the hospital room, a somber choir in silent lamentation. It was imperative no one weep, since the person who is dying is the one who has the most right to be upset and if they're managing to keep it together, who are we to let our tears flow in their presence? Breathing deeply, I tried to steady myself. Dad emerged from the room, face drained. It was my turn.

Nothing in life prepares you to be present at someone's deathbed. But my mother was seated in a chair! She had not been out of bed in a week and this involved a colossal effort. She willed herself to be chipper (how was this possible?) and watched as I settled into a chair opposite. Her hair wispy now; her face sunken and gray. Thoughts of her skiing, playing tennis, riding her bike through leafy suburban streets, sun-dappled and quiet, making sandwiches, giving rides, drinking coffee, and talking. Always present.

A few months earlier she had attended a party at our apartment. In a swirl of chatter and bonhomie, I looked up and caught a glimpse of her alone in the hall outside the room absorbing the lively scene before she drifted off, the empty doorway a premonition.

She thanked me for being a good son—at that moment all vexations forgotten—and said some other words my neural pathways were too scrambled to recall. Not really knowing how to respond, I immediately apologized for anything I ever did that had exasperated her or made her angry. She smiled wanly, shook her head as if to say *don't be ridiculous.* I used to be able to make my mother laugh, great rollicking guffaws that shook her entire body. Dad would look at her like she was crazy; he never thought what I'd said was that funny.

Despite my ability to make her lose control, we did not have a relationship where I could do no wrong. I've done the requisite number of ill-considered things and she was aware of some of them. She made her displeasure known. We had our arguments and sometimes they were loud. She was my first boundary and, in some ways, remained my best one. In the aftermath of anything I wasn't supposed to be doing, I wondered what she would say if she knew: hence, the default apology. But mostly I was filling the air since I had no idea what to say. I scrutinized every word or phrase that arose in my consciousness and all of them felt insufficient. The minutes ticked away. An intense and unforeseen helplessness overcame me. Death demands acceptance from those witnessing it and acceptance is something with which human beings in these liminal spaces are penurious.

When I was five years old and couldn't swim, I drifted from the shallow end of a swimming pool to where the water was over my head. Because my feet could not touch the bottom, I was unable to get back to the shallow end. I thrashed and yelled, struggling and failing to keep my head above water. My mother was nearby, on a chaise. Fully dressed, she leaped into the pool. Picture her suspended in the summer air over shimmering blue water, rippling with life.

After four years of fighting, through which she carried herself with dignity and intermittent humor, my mother died on a September afternoon. She was sixty-one, two years younger than I am now. It was a year and a day after our wedding. Susan and I had gone for a walk, thinking nothing was imminent. We arrived back in the room at two o'clock and saw that her breathing, which had been even, had become inconsistent. My father and brother were at the bedside. I sat next to Dad and took her hand, shocked, immobile. Tell her you love her, he said. I rose to my feet, leaned close, and whispered those words into her ear. A doctor once told me that when a person is dying their hearing is the last sense to go. It's impossible to know whether or not she heard my words but there was comfort in that it was not the first time I'd said them to her. Now she struggled, face tense. Her chest rose slightly with each intake of air. This went on for nearly fifteen minutes. And then it didn't. Her body relaxed and her eyes were wide open, facing the ceiling. Her face paled. She looked beatific, a Renaissance painting of a saint. She wasn't a saint. Who is, aside from Richard Nixon's mother, and that's according to Nixon, an unreliable narrator. And all of the certified Catholic saints. But not my mother, who liked her martinis very, very dry.

Now she was gone. Dad stood over her and quietly said, I'll meet you on the Riviera.

Bix and Brooke ride again.

I thought: *If only.*

We packed up the room. I kissed her still-warm forehead and

thought about the times as a child when I would come into my parents' room to talk to them before bedtime. My mother slept on the side of the bed near the door so that's where I would sit. We would talk about what I had done that day, what I might be worried about, what I had planned. Now I looked over my right shoulder as I left the room and saw my mother lying in bed for the last time. There are people, I'm told, who view death as a great adventure. There is no one like that in our family.

The four of us, my father, my brother, Susan, and I visited the now conveniently located Riverside Memorial Chapel to select a casket and make the funeral arrangements. Then we went upstairs to our apartment for dinner since none of us could bear to be alone.

At our wedding, the photographer was so distracted he failed to get a picture of my family with Susan and me. This troubled my mother so over Thanksgiving she summoned him back to take a family portrait. We all squeezed back into our formal gear and posed in front of the fireplace at my parents' house. But the photographer must have been distracted again because when we saw the result, I wished he had never taken the picture. He had lit us badly and my mother, on the left of the frame, was edged in darkness.

In the Uffizi Gallery in Florence there hang side by side three self-portraits by Rembrandt. In each he is progressively older; brightly lit in the first, shadowed in the second, and in the third it is as if the artist is being swallowed by eternity.

My mother framed the family photograph and gave us each a copy.

At the time of her death, I was amazed by the recent trend of people speaking at funerals. I did not understand this at all. Now that I've done it a few times, I'm more accustomed to the idea but back then it was like wing-walking. In those days, if anyone to whom I was close died, I was in no condition to speak in public. Writing an essay about them is one thing, but the idea of saying the words aloud put marbles in my mouth. I was in awe of people who could speak eloquently at a funeral, but they lived in another emotional universe.

I wrote a eulogy. It consisted of several interlinked stories, all intended to convey my mother's pluck. My favorite: she was a terrible skier and as a result fell down a lot. One winter day years ago, I looked out the kitchen window toward our snow-covered backyard. There she was on skis, in her familiar seated position. When I asked her what she was doing she informed me that she was practicing getting up.

People like to hear the inspirational stuff, particularly when faced with death, since it gives them hope that perhaps within their own breast there is a bit of indomitability, too.

The day before the funeral Dad gave me a journal my mother kept the year before her death. It was the Chronicle of a Nightmare. Each entry revealed she was hoping for a little good news but none ever came. She bargained with God for more time. She prayed to her dead mother. Her greatest wish was to live long enough for my daughter to remember her. In her journal, she wrote that she wanted to carry herself in such a way so that when she died, no one would be relieved. No one was relieved. The depression, pain, and longing in its pages made it agonizing to read but the spirit that animated her days shone through. It was like reading the *Diary of Anne Frank* if Anne was my mother. You love the character, the reality of her lived experience is indelible as is her mettle, and you know something terrible is going to happen.

My parents had joined a suburban synagogue in their later years, and this is where the service was to be held. We selected a colorful Marimekko dress in which my mother would be buried and when I saw her in the coffin I was surprised by how good she looked, particularly under the circumstances. I kissed her forehead, which had grown cold in the intervening days, and suddenly realized she had spent them in a refrigerator. This is the curious duality one becomes aware of at a funeral. The corpse is there, but the person is absent. An obvious enough idea, but it is comforting when you are assaulted by thoughts like *my mother has been in a refrigerator*. No, in fact she has *not* been in a refrigerator. Her *body*, the abandoned worldly envelope, the vessel through which her spirit traversed the earth has but *she* has not. A small but nonetheless reassuring distinction. An exchange occurred at my maternal grandmother's funeral when I was fourteen that brought this home early. My brother, our cousin Miles, and I were at the funeral home on Queens Boulevard chatting about the Mets' pennant chances when Miles's mother approached and asked if he wanted to see Grandma.

Oh, he replied, is she here?

The service for my mother took place and because I was too much of a coward to speak in public given my fragile emotional state the rabbi read my eulogy. I am retrospectively embarrassed by this but history is undeniable. There were no other speakers. I wore sunglasses since I could not put a bag over my head.

There was a receiving line in the temple library after the service, where people offered condolences, and these moments were difficult since they have a this-is-your-life quality. People I had not seen in years shook my hand, murmured commiseration, and tried to impart something that cannot be communicated in words. They looked older and I looked older; everyone sailing toward the distant shore. The burial ceremony was brief, the prayers almost all in Hebrew, a language I do not speak more than a few words of. It was gray, drizzling, and I thought of the old Elmore James lyric—*The sky is crying, look at the tears roll down the street*. Dad shoveled earth on the casket, then I did, then Drew. As soon as the graveside service ended, I slanted through the crowd of mourners, settled into the car, and let tears arrive, something to which I had become alarmingly accustomed.

Friends and family descended on my parents' house (it was hard to think of it as anything other than that even though it was now my father's house) after the funeral to drink and eat. Gazing around: *This looks like a party but the hostess is dead.* It was not as if everyone should be keening, ululating, rending garments, but something was missing. Oh, for the Vikings and their burning boats, and the flaming pyres of India, into which the occasional bereaved spouse would dive in hopes of following their beloved to the afterlife, Tibetan sky burials where monks place a body on a platform exposed to nature and the vultures do the rest, basic, primal rituals that speak to the essence of death. These were societies that understood what was required. My Great Aunt Gussie from Cleveland by way of Ukraine launched herself on my paternal grandmother's coffin in a paroxysm of grief. *That* was more like it. Grandma and Aunt Gussie had been born in Europe and traveled to America as young girls. Once here, they both struggled to make ends meet and now one of them was lying in a coffin in a funeral home on Queens Boulevard. Great Aunt Gussie was justifiably upset. Her display may not have involved fires or predatory birds but it broke through the forced decorum of the modern death experience. The ritual of nibbling cake and sipping coffee felt inadequate to the moment. I considered the possibility that my mother's death was not being experienced on a deep enough level, although I found myself dreading nightfall.

Whenever our family went to a restaurant my mother had to change her table at least twice. It was too near the kitchen, or the restrooms, or there was a draft. It got so that we would wait until she had finished playing musical chairs and only then all move to her final selection. Before she got sick, I would always kid her, joking, At your funeral, you're going to sit up in the coffin and say, I want to be over there.

Not long after the funeral I received a phone call from Dad. "I think they buried Mom facing the wrong direction."

"Excuse me?" I was at the graveside. I witnessed the casket being lowered into the ground. I shoveled ceremonial dirt. Facing the wrong direction? This could not be right. "Are you sure?"

"Her feet are under the headstone."

"She's backwards?"

This was—unexpected. My mother was a stickler for correct form and facing the wrong direction for eternity would not have pleased her. The gulf of years between then and now allows for an acknowledgment of the irony. But at the time, despite having a chiaroscuro sense of humor, the comic side of my mother's prospective exhumation eluded me. The notion of excavating her coffin just so we could make sure it had been correctly placed in the grave was seriously—*off*. Once you interred someone they were meant to stay in the ground. It occurred to me that the problem my father was experiencing was not the direction in which my mother was buried; rather, it was that she was *buried*.

A few days passed and then, while we were having lunch in a restaurant near his office, Dad mentioned it again.

"I think they buried Mom facing the wrong direction."

"I know. That's what you said. Listen, you're upset," I pointed out. "That's a pretty major mistake so I think it's unlikely."

He nodded and went back to his ravioli. A week went by. We were at his weekend house. Standing in the kitchen, he looked me directly in the eye and said, "Seth, I can't stop thinking about it. I called the Rabbi. We're going to dig her up."

Dig her up?

The Rabbi informed my father that, yes, there was a prayer

for this occasion and he would be pleased to stand by the grave and recite it. Apparently, it was not the first time in Jewish history something like this had occurred. My brother and I were ambivalent about the disinterment but it had become a fixation for Dad and we had no choice but to go along. This was not a ship I was steering; if our father wanted to exhume our mother's grave there was not much to do other than offer support. He was right to make sure. Humankind devised the idea of ceremony as a means of creating order in a chaotic world. Burials are the last chance the living are given to bestow harmony upon the memory of the dead. Now my mother's burial had become some kind of ghoulish routine, Laurel and Hardy by way of Edgar Allan Poe. But we would be sure it had been done correctly and if it had not, the blunder would be rectified.

Under a reproving sky, Dad, Drew, Susan, and I stood with the Rabbi as the workmen dug up the grave. A stoical representative from Riverside Memorial Chapel hovered nearby wishing—I'm certain—that he was anywhere but here. How could it be that the gravediggers, who had *one job*, would get it so egregiously wrong? It was as if the dentist drilled your elbow. Not something that would happen. We made conversation and tried to ignore the preposterous nature of the event. Like a film running in reverse, out flew the dirt, rising in a soft pile to the side of the grave. Ten, twenty, thirty minutes passed while they finished. Finally, with great trepidation we all peered down.

The dentist had drilled the elbow.

At that point we retreated to position fifty feet from the grave and huddled together, newly shocked and still grief stricken. How does something like this occur? It is a simple enough job, grave digging. Dig a hole. Make sure the casket's facing the right way. Place the casket in the hole. A three-item checklist, not exactly splitting the atom.

And yet.

Events we don't remotely anticipate keep happening.

The workmen climbed into the grave—was this the crack team that had done the burial?—and dexterously ran straps beneath the coffin. Then they proceeded to hoist it into the air and turn it around. It was a great relief they did not drop it. Seeing my mother's coffin lifted from the earth less than a month after we had buried her was wildly disorienting, the world tipping out of alignment. We forced ourselves to watch only to be certain it was done correctly the second time.

The representative from Riverside, a thin, balding man in a dark suit, turned to Dad and said, "Sorry for the inconvenience." Oh, it's no inconvenience, I remember thinking. We're just digging up my dead mother.

*I don't like where we're sitting. Let's change tables.*

Grief is fluid, malleable. It can become anger or rage quickly, before reverting to deep sadness. I thought my father might kill him but instead we went to a restaurant. The hostess led the three of us to a table and there we remained.

\* \* \*

Autumn passed uneventfully but Thanksgiving was askew the year my mother died. It was always her holiday. She cooked for days and an extended family of aunts, uncles, cousins, and friends would descend on our house. No one wanted to do Thanksgiving that year but my father soldiered on.

Three generations of relatives came.

We played touch football.

It all felt wrong.

Then it was the Season of Joy.

I was looking forward to Christmas even less than usual, because in 1991 I hated Christmas. This was not always the case. As a small child, Christmas envy ruled. I wanted a tree with presents under it and plum pudding. I didn't know what plum pudding was; but if it was Christmas-related, it had to be good. Christmas had nothing to do with Jesus. I hadn't even heard of Jesus when I loved Christmas. It was snow, and sleighs, and gaily wrapped gifts. I loved Christmas at a time when you could use the word *gaily* in a sentence without thinking twice. At my public school, we sang Christmas carols. This was not negotiable. There was no Hanukkah music provided for us, no "I Had a Little Dreidel" song sheets passed out to counterbalance the torrent of relentlessly joyful and seductive Christmas music. During the holiday season in Scarsdale it was all Christmas all the time and if the Jews had a problem, they could send their kids to yeshivas. Not only did this blatant attempt to jam Christmas down our throats in a tax-funded setting not bother me, I embraced it, belted the carols with enthusiasm, dreamed those sugarplum dreams. And when my parents told me in no uncertain terms that a Christmas tree was a nonstarter, I felt persecuted. I had a Jewish friend whose parents succumbed to the prevailing mythos and placed a dwarfish tree on a credenza in their living room. My friend was very proud of this tinseled bush, although it struck me as a sad half-measure.

My parents refused to budge from the no-tree edict. Year after year they held firm. We would have our eight nights of Hanukkah, all of us gathered around the menorah, my brother and me in our pajamas, opening gifts, bathed in the light of the candles. I loved Hanukkah. But the existential emptiness that descended when Christmas morning arrived in our treeless and undecorated living room was profound. This feeling ended with my childhood and by the time I was in my twenties and living in Manhattan, Christmas came to mean Chinese food and a movie.

But this holiday season found me in Paw Paw, Michigan, Susan's hometown, for Christmas on Mars. Paw Paw is situated on I-94 exactly halfway between 1961 and 1962. A quintessential midwestern small town, it's comprised of a Main Street, lots of churches, and, on the spur leading to the Interstate, every fast food restaurant you can think of.

There were no Jews.

When I went to Paw Paw the Jewish population soared by 100%. I became a one-man production of *Fiddler on the Roof*, the receptacle and representative of Spinoza and Maimonides, a nose with two legs. I was the first Jew a lot of these people had met. I sensed them looking for my horns, which I had the foresight to hide under a loose-fitting hat.

Early in our visit I was seated at the kitchen table in my sister-in-law Catie's house, conveniently down the road from the house Susan grew up in and where her parents still lived. Hearty and loquacious, my sister-in-law was a friendly midwestern woman; we liked each other. The two of us were drinking soda from cans.

In the most benevolent tone imaginable, she said, "I just don't understand how a person can't accept that Jesus is our savior." By the third evening I had been there for a year. When Christmas finally arrived, I retired from the festivities and spent the day in bed reading Paul Johnson's *A History of the Jews*. This did not make Susan's day easier.

\* \* \*

Six weeks after the Christmas at which my sister-in-law implied that my eternal soul was in peril if I did not accept her cosmology, I learned that my nearly seventy-two-year-old father was dating a demanding and volatile thirty-eight-year-old Brazilian Catholic woman who claimed to be a close friend of Cardinal O'Connor. You would be forgiven for thinking he had met her on the way home from my mother's funeral. They actually met at a Manhattan clothier where she was trawling for sugar daddies from her perch behind the counter. She sold him shirts. He bought several.

The signal word that ruled my mother's life was *appropriate*. It was the lens through which she viewed the world. Something was appropriate, or not; the categories were immutable. She dressed appropriately, behaved appropriately; venerated the concept of *appropriateness*. It wasn't always the easiest trait to digest when I was growing up because our views of what was appropriate occasionally diverged. In my childhood, on special occasions, she would dress my brother and me in blue blazers and saddle shoes. The blue blazer was trouble enough, but the saddle shoes were humiliating to my nascent sense of fashion. To my mother, however, they were the height of appropriate. Why she wanted us to look like we were going to a lawn party at the Duke of Buckingham's country house in 1937 was a mystery, but it was non-negotiable.

When I was a freshman in high school a six-foot-high, psychedelic poster of Jim Morrison screamed from my bedroom wall. It was a Blakean vision, a hallucinatory image designed to frighten people like my mother into thinking any fourteen-year-old who displayed it was five minutes from dropping acid and decamping to Haight-Ashbury to play music, have indiscriminate sex, and not bathe—all of which, admittedly, held a certain appeal at the time. She felt the poster was *inappropriate*. That I found it to be the very essence of appropriate did not matter. Here is how the scene went, and I will apologize in advance for the lack of subtlety with the explanation that the era in which the scene occurred was unsubtle:

*Time: 1969*
*Dramatis personae:*
*My mother, 39 years old.*
*Me, 14.*
*Setting: A suburban teenage boy's room. I am lying on a*

*single bed staring at the ceiling. My mother enters. She will
live another twenty-two years, although neither of us know
this at the time. A large poster of Jim Morrison, who has
recently been found dead in a Parisian bathtub, catches her
eye. He looks positively Mephistophelean and my mother's
hair stands on end.*
Mother: *You have to take that poster down.*
Me: *No.*
Mother: *I said you have to take that poster down.*
Me: *And I said no. And why should I? It's an expression
of who I am.*
Mother: *You're a kid from the suburbs!*
Me: *On the surface, maybe. But there's a whole lot more
going on, Mom. Maybe I can't let my freak flag fly because
you won't let me, but Jim Morrison is under no such con-
straints and I intend to keep this mind-blowing six-foot rendering of his depraved face here on my wall forever no matter what anyone says!*
Mother: *Take that poster down or I'm going to get your
father to come in here.*
*(She stares at me. I stare back. She stares. I stare back. She
stares. I blink.)*
*CURTAIN*

When my mother wanted to exert control, the invocation of
*your father* never failed to work. In his early years, my father was
usually agreeable but his wrath, once awakened, was intense.
Like a tornado, it wasn't something you wanted to experience
twice. Down came Jim Morrison in all his purple-eyed,
gold-flamed hair, peyote-fueled glory. Rolled up and placed in
the closet where he rested beneath my jeans and flannel shirts.
We didn't always agree. Still, she influenced me, and twenty-
two years later this bossa nova romance of Dad's felt inappropriate. It makes me sound a tad priggish, I know. Starchy,

straitlaced; qualities we can agree to abhor. Stipulated: better he should enjoy himself than weep into a bottle of gin. But his choice of companion was problematic and Susan and Drew seconded this assessment. It was challenging enough that she was my age. That was unfortunate but didn't disqualify her. She had no money, wanted to be a writer despite never having written anything, and displayed an impressive devotion to whiskey which was probably not unrelated to her occasionally turning up in the lobby of Dad's apartment building tipsy and uninvited at 4:00 A.M. The whole farrago read like a discarded draft of an unpublished Theodore Dreiser novel. But whenever a struggling young woman takes up with an older man of means, the scent of grifting is in the air. And here's what was really troubling: her husband was a hairdresser who had recently died of AIDS. As a package, the downside was considerable. This is not to disparage hairdressers or people with AIDS. That this woman might have exchanged bodily fluids with someone who had died from a disease that had wiped out a considerable proportion of lower Manhattan was not just a warning signal but more like the wild semaphores of a Ritalin swilling five-year-old.

Unleashed from thirty-five years of monogamy, arthritic hormones suddenly rampaging like Godzilla through downtown Tokyo, my father was willing to roll the dice. He got an AIDS test. If you have never experienced your recently widowed parent announcing the results of the AIDS test he took because he is dating an emotionally unstable Brazilian woman your own age whose dead husband was a hairdresser, the words that spring to mind to describe the resulting sensation are *cognitive dissonance* along with some other less gracious ones. Every time we got together I yelled at him—she's unstable, she's after your money, do you even know her immigration status, she probably wants to marry you for a green card—but he was so pleased with himself he would just laugh and laugh.

Like it was funny, which to him it was. He was a widower lacerated with grief into whose lap the universe had placed a nubile younger woman, albeit one with serious psychological issues (she would eventually threaten suicide if he refused her bidding), and said *I dare you.*

And his response: *Oh, really? Watch this!*

Liberated from doctors' offices, hospital room vigils, cancer, and imminent death, he rose like an amorous phoenix and proudly beat his wings. Once, after one of my lectures, he responded by doing a little dance that consisted of pretending to climb an invisible ladder while singing a ditty whose only lyrics consisted of *fuckee, fuck-ah, fuckee, fuck-ah . . .*

A genuine fertility dance, and if it wasn't exactly the kind you study in a college anthropology class, it was a first cousin. He was celebrating not being dead. As an example of the life force, this was admirable. Alan Arkin will play him in the movie. But despite the troubled path he was merrily gamboling down (*fuckee, fuck-ah, fuckee, fuck-ah*), nothing could dissuade him and I eventually concluded my father, while unhinged by sorrow, was indefatigable, which was positive, and tried to let it rest. I avoided meeting the woman.

Then I encountered her at a party.

Early evening in an Upper East Side apartment. Drinks and hors d'oeuvres. A compact, olive-skinned minx surged toward me on spiked heels, attractive features angrily flaring. In a matching purple tweed skirt and jacket, she had fierce brown eyes, lipstick the color of blood, and abundant black hair that swept past histrionic shoulders.

"I love your father," she spat. "Don't get in our way."

Someone was not playing the subtext. Apparently, Dad had conveyed to her my reservations about their budding relationship, which made me the obstacle.

"Good to finally meet you," I lied. Telenovela was not a language I spoke.

"I love him," she repeated, in case I had missed it the first time. The reiteration was more belligerent. Her shoulders levitated. This lady wanted to rumble.

Observing the crowded room, it was obvious to me that escalation was not an option, so I nodded with feigned understanding. Staring up at me fists clenched, she held her ground for several uncomfortable seconds but after her initial thrust had been met with a temperate response, there was nothing for her to work with and our exchange fizzled as quickly as it had begun. This is what my father likes? Her ferocious bearing so unsettled me that I soon left the party, Susan bewildered in my wake.

A week later I was in Los Angeles on business. While there, Dad's new girlfriend called our apartment repeatedly and hung up as soon as Susan answered. This behavior went on for several hours, deep into the night. Then it happened again, another night. We changed our phone number. We complained to Dad. He did not believe it was her. And why should he have? He was reliving an unbridled version of his youth and did not want to be tethered to reality.

\* \* \*

After experiencing my daughter's birth, my mother's death, and the disorientation of my father's bereavement fling, I found myself at the NYU Medical Center taking a doctor-ordered stress test. Perhaps I was fated not to take after my rejuvenated father, whose veins currently coursed with molten lava, but my maternal grandfather of the eleven heart attacks. A razor-wielding nurse shaved the chest hair that has thwarted my career as an underwear model and placed electrodes on my ribs. These would be connected to a machine that was going to record my heart rate as I walked briskly on a treadmill and tried not to think about what had landed me in this position. Standing barefoot on the gray linoleum of the hallway holding the handful of wires protruding from my chest, another nurse appeared and announced I had a phone call. I froze. Anyone who tracks you down at a hospital where you're having a stress test is not calling with good news.

"Seth, it's Drew. This is not good news."

Immediately, I thought our father had expired, probably *in flagrante*, which would have made a certain amount of sense. Then I thought something happened to Susan. Then I thought—

"Susan's brother died."

*Excuse me?*

One of the ways Aristotle defines tragedy is that it be surprising, yet inevitable. This development neatly fit the bill. Susan's brother was thirty-eight and alcoholic. Heart failure.

Stripped the wires, got dressed, cabbed to our apartment. There I found my wife collapsed in a heap of the blackest misery. Susan had been close with her brother in childhood. Sensitive kids, natural allies. They'd grown slowly apart as their lives took radically different trajectories but now that he was gone it was ripping her heart out. My brother-in-law Bill died in Minneapolis and his body had to be brought to Paw Paw for the funeral. Five hours later we were on a plane to Michigan.

The family had a visitation at the funeral home and it was every bit as sad as a gathering for someone who was thirty-eight years old and has died should be. Susan's sister was there, and her parents, uncles, and aunts. Tommy McNeil, a crony of Bill's, a formerly hard-partying guy who knew it could have been he in the casket, cornered Susan and me, telling us how the Lord saved him from drink. Tommy had tried to sell Bill on the good word but Bill hadn't been buying. There was a healthy crowd at the early show (2:00–4:00) and an even better one at the late show (7:00–9:00). People never paid this much attention when he was alive.

At the funeral home, there was a group prayer where everyone in the family stood in a circle holding hands—Susan and her sister, her father and mother, aunts, uncles, and me.

*Our Father who art in Heaven, hallowed be thy name—*

Everything was smooth sailing until my Catholic father-in-law and his equally Catholic sisters started with the Hail Marys. Holy Mary, Mother of—*Mother*! Catholic, Muslim, Jewish, it didn't matter, mother is mother in every language and that was when I disintegrated, reliving my mother's too-recent, too early death, thinking—so moved was I by this prayer—perhaps I was Catholic in a former life, if I believed in past lives, which I do not. But there is something alarmingly visceral about Catholicism besides the centuries of magnificent if blood-drenched art it inspired. The rituals the major religious have devised to mark the passing of their adherents abide for good reason. I choked back sobs and got on with listening to the prayer.

*Holy Mary, Mother of God, pray for us sinners now and at the hour of our death.*

The next day Reverend Lumm, a bearded Presbyterian of elfish aspect who were he a few inches shorter would not have been out of place in Tolkien's Shire, conducted a fine funeral service that praised the dead and solaced the living. Since Bill was a photographer, he seized on the metaphor and alluded to how lives sometimes get out of focus.

I gained five pounds that week by going on the Mourner's Diet which consists of gorging on everything placed in front of you six times a day. Even though I barely knew Bill, I was already wrung out, so it was a struggle to not let his death knock me off my perilous equilibrium. Having recently endured the mourning process, such a quick return trip was unwelcome. But I was mindful of Susan and her experience. Mostly, I thought about her parents. How could they survive this?

The family plot was twelve hours north in the Upper

Peninsula of Michigan and we dutifully flew up there and laid Bill to rest.

But not in the earth.

At least not yet.

He was placed in storage. Since the ground was frozen and they can't dig graves until the thaw, the dead are filed away like old letters until springtime. You hope they're buried facing the right direction.

There was a graveside service on a frigid northern Michigan day which answered the family's need for finality. The wind swirled under gray skies as we shivered among the monuments, Catholics buried on one side of the rolling field, Protestants on the other, divided by doctrine (and a narrow road), united in death where all Christians are equal and believe they will ascend to an agreed-upon Heaven where no one will ever have to take a stress test.

\* \* \*

In my younger and less vulnerable years, when death seemed as distant as the Aurora Borealis, I asked my father what our family believed happens when someone died. He thought about it for a moment and said:

"We live on in the hearts of those who knew us."

"There's no Heaven?"

"It's all right here," he said, indicating our den. A couch, a television, a bookshelf, a sleeping dog, and a fireplace. My shoulders slumped. I was maybe twelve.

Over the next few decades, I did not much consider the prospect of an afterlife because I refused to believe I might be going there any time soon. And when I was diagnosed with cancer, I didn't think about it because I convinced myself I was not going to die at that time. But having managed to grow older, I've been contemplating available roadmaps. Allow me to proceed with the caveat that I am not a religious scholar so what follows reflects a hobbyist's interest. And for the sake of concision, let's agree to leave the specifics of Hell for another time.

The seventy-two virgins promised to Islamic martyrs aside (And, really, what kind of lunatic would actually want to be confronted by seventy-two virgins?), it's easy to conclude that Christians tell the simplest and most superficially appealing post-death story as far as what happens to the believer who is not sent to Hell or the Hell equivalent. Different branches have divergent ideas about how divine real estate is apportioned—the waiting room known as Purgatory for example, where dead souls are stuck until their fate is adjudicated, is a Roman Catholic idea eschewed by mainstream Protestantism—but they're all singing from the same hymnal about Heaven: a gauzy mirror of life on Earth with more reliable weather.

Less well known than the mainstream iteration of Christian Heaven is the Mormon version. There is some disagreement among Mormons themselves about what happens when one of their number expires. Do they dwell in the shadow of God on the planet Kolob? Or do they get their own personal planet? Church elders eventually settled upon a concept of Heaven divided into three realms. The top level is the Celestial Kingdom, a resplendent domain of unimaginable glory. The middle level is the Terrestrial Kingdom, which has some glory, but not that much. And the bottom level is the Telestial Kingdom, which to an observant Mormon must feel like landing in public housing. So while Mormons are technically Christian, their Heaven has a ghetto.

Certain modern practitioners of Christianity welcome the Enlightenment notion that the doctrines pertaining to Heaven are meant to be taken as metaphor, but great swaths of Christendom continue to believe that Heaven is an actual place where they will be reunited with dead relatives. That this idea has persisted for two millennia flies in the face of family dynamics as we know them in the modern world where to some, being reunited with their family for eternity is a fate more befitting the souls that have been remitted to Hell. But for the kind of person who is able to ignore that she hasn't spoken to one of her sisters since the fight last Christmas over who put vodka in the children's eggnog, it remains a popular notion.

The Christian idea of Heaven held great appeal. The prospect of seeing my parents and grandparents again was enough to get me to try and forestall assignment to wherever the metaphysical authorities send pretentious masturbators who never learned to properly play the piano or speak more than rudimentary French despite taking it for more than *six years* in school because I would actually *want* to see my dead relatives. This doesn't mean that I would want to see them every day for all of eternity, but a family dinner in some warm corner of the cosmos without the pressure of occasion-driven gift giving would be welcome.

This kind of mystical event would not be possible in the Buddhist tradition where shuffling offstage is easier said than done. There are three major branches of Buddhism, Theravada, Mahayana, and Vajrayana, and predictably, because nothing unites practitioners of a religion more than the inability to agree on anything, they have a different view of what happens when we die. They do, however, agree on the goal: Nirvana, the state one reaches after successive rounds of reincarnation during which the essence of the departed—Buddhists do not believe in a permanent soul—attempts to perfect itself in a new incarnation. This cycle of day-to-day life is known by the Sanskrit word samsara and liberation from samsara is the Buddhist equivalent of the search for an affordable apartment on Central Park West.

Why do Buddhist practitioners want to be liberated from samsara? Because it represents the uprooting of greed, hatred, and delusion. And the desire for liberation is easy to understand if you think of the Buddhist view of life and death as the equivalent of climbing a mountain in the rain with a filing cabinet strapped to your back, reaching the summit, then being told by whatever determines your fate—universal consciousness? A monk in the back office?—that you didn't get it quite right, so please go back to the bottom of the mountain and do it again in a new body, without your previous knowledge, but with all of your karma which, too bad for you, was not good enough to attain Nirvana, so better luck next time, move along, you're holding up the line. The metaphysical arena between worldly incarnations where this takes place is what's known in the Tibetan tradition as the Bardo, and it's similar to the Christian concept of purgatory, a way station. While Christians believe the living can pray for dead souls stuck in purgatory, in the Bardo you're on your own. No one wants to remain in the Bardo. It's like waiting for the F train on a lonely platform in the middle of the night. During a transit strike. As for getting out of samsara, this seems like trying to escape a prison riot. Does anyone achieve Nirvana? Who knows? Let's assume someone does—and this is key to understanding how the Buddhist concept of the afterlife differs from the Judeo-Christian one: individual subjective identity ceases to exist because in the Buddhist view life is suffering and suffering is caused by clinging to things, and not just things like sex or a beach house or eyeglass frames that are actually flattering to your face, but things like an individual identity. Arguably, there are living Buddhists who have uprooted greed, hatred, and delusion, and achieved Nirvana here on Earth. I've never met one but if I did I would buy her a drink and toast the accomplishment.

To my western mind, the Buddhist afterlife is, like the gourmet cheeseburger, an irresolvable paradox. One labors through end-less incarnations, evolving and purifying, and rather than being able to reap the rewards of all of that karmic improvement, the prize is the dissolution of whatever it was that constituted "you" as an individual. Of course, if "you're" a Buddhist, that's the point.

When I recently began to reassess the exceedingly vaporous metaphysical condominium of "the hearts of those who knew you" with which I was raised and where my father informed me we would live on, it still struck me as weak tea and, depending on my view of death at the moment I was cog-itating on the "hearts" idea, could unleash a set of feelings ranging from disappointing to petrifying. But is it weak tea? Or a concept incumbent upon any rational person to finally accept.

Because Jews of all stripes tend to be focused on the tem-poral world, there is not a lot of afterlife-related dogma, which leaves space for eccentric ideas to take root. This comforting rabbinic bunkum was denied me. Later, I learned there are Jews who believe in all kinds of afterlife-related esoterica. The Jewish afterlife is called Olam Ha-Ba which translates as the World to Come and when the Messiah finally arrives dead souls will be resurrected and dwell there for eternity. No con-sensus exists about what this place is actually like so there is lots of room for individual projection. To me, this vitiates the entire endeavor because if you can interpret it however you wish, it takes what is a fantasy to begin with and only further muddies the waters. Also, the notion that "the Jews" could ever possibly agree on the identity of the Messiah? Two Jews, three opinions, goes the popular (for a reason) adage.

There are Orthodox Jews who believe virtuous souls go to a place similar to the Christian heaven, although presumably without any Christians or secular Jews. A strain of Orthodox thought embraces reincarnation, which might get to the root of the affinity certain Jews have for Buddhism. The Kabbalists are fervent believers in the transmigration of souls and highly imaginative about their manifestations. The soul of a pompous fool upon death will enter the body of a cockroach until he atones for whatever led to his bad behavior (how a cockroach engages with the concept of atonement is a question better left to the rabbis). The folkloric Dybbuk is a tormented soul pursued by demons who takes refuge in a human body and must be exorcised. As for the Hasidim, practitioners of ecstatic worship, they love the idea of reincarnation almost as much as they love dancing with other men. All of which makes me wonder why reincarnation did not make it into the mainstream of Jewish life where it could have done so much in the way of softening the harsh blow that knowledge of the terminal nature of existence represents for most people.

What unifies all cosmic visions of the afterlife is the idea of solace in the present and hope for a radiant future in the light of eternity. And perhaps most powerfully, the potential absence of fear. If there is something more primal than the fear of death, I'm not sure what it is, and it is this bug in the human genome that drives much of the religious enterprise. It is one of the reasons that despite the hectoring of clever atheists religion will always abide.

It will be a great surprise to me if it turns out that there is a hereafter where I am sentient. I have made no plans to be sentient and would find that eternity spent working out my various psychological issues enervating. Perhaps there exists a version where one's neuroses miraculously vanish somewhere in the space-time continuum, but that idea seems even more implausible than the galactic tub of butter where we get to be a better edition of who we were on Earth.

After the events of 9/11 the professional football player Pat Tillman enlisted in the army. He became a Ranger and was subsequently killed in Afghanistan. Senator John McCain eulogized him at the funeral and said, He's in a better place, to which Pat Tillman's brother replied: No he's not. He's fucking dead.

My father was right. Heaven was our family home the day I inquired about the afterlife. It's connection. Tenderness. Joy. I am not a sojourner traveling toward an ultimate realm. This is where I live.

\* \* \*

Upon our return to New York after Bill's funeral, we put our suitcases down and looked at each other.

"What next?" I said.

Susan replied: "I'm pregnant."

The timing was too perfect. Were this a novel, an editor would advise the author to slow down, there's too much plot, too many events. But this was not a novel. Life was intruding immediately upon death, insisting on its primacy. And all right, a little soon, but nothing the two of us couldn't handle. We had been dealing with a lot of emotionally fraught developments. But we wanted another kid so if this was the timing, it would have to work. At the window of our living room, staring into the Manhattan darkness, life felt like a Russian novel, birth, death, and infinity on every page.

The following month Susan had a miscarriage.

This was piling on. Yes, there are villages in Africa whose suffering is exponentially greater. Worse things happen to millions of people. But this trifecta of unhappiness was nonetheless emotionally devastating and left us bludgeoned. You're going along, and going along, and everything is fine. And then it isn't. And isn't again. And then isn't one more time, and how much can a person take?

Some people believe death arrives in groups of three. If this is true, then it was almost predictable. Susan dealt with it as well as a person can deal with something so ghastly and primal. I barely had the mental capacity to think about it. Still reeling from my mother's death, the early pregnancy was too abstract. Bill's passing added to the general emotional lassitude prevalent at the time. These are excuses of which I'm not proud. The ability to handle this succession of calamities other than perfunctorily was not there. It was one more in a litany of Job-like experiences that had become our two-mules-yoked-to-a-plow lot. There wasn't much talk about it. What was there to say other than death was all around, hovering, ubiquitous, poised to fly through the window at any moment, dark wings whipping, and take someone else away?

And we already knew that.

In the summer of the year Bill died we went back to Michigan to visit Susan's family. They were in Calumet in the Upper Peninsula, a weatherworn, beaten down place on the decline since the copper mining companies pulled up stakes eighty years ago. The town as hollowed out as we felt. Sixth Street, the main drag, resembled a hockey player's teeth. Most of the young people were gone and the ones who remained looked like they'd been arrested for operating a snowmobile while intoxicated.

Bill had been buried that spring, when the ground had thawed. His passing was like a weather front, heavy and stultifying. The family burial plot was two miles from their summer home, the dead ever present. Susan's parents visited his grave often. Bill's death was doubly hard on them because they mourned the wreck of his life while he was living; and now that he was dead, they mourned that. My father-in-law, not a particularly devout man, listened to Catholic mass on the radio, which made Susan cry. The atmosphere was unrelentingly funereal.

When we returned to New York I learned Jim Valvano had bone cancer and it had spread to his sneakers. He was a young basketball coach who led North Carolina State to an improbable national championship in 1983. Drew and I had watched Valvano's victory together in my small Los Angeles apartment. When the buzzer sounded, he ran around the court jumping up and down, hugging everyone he could get his hands on. That long-ago night he looked like a man who would live forever.

The following week was my thirty-seventh birthday. The tang of middle age in the air. The days and weeks shot past at a numbing pace. Then, writer's block. Words came out, prolixity was not the problem. I was skating along the surface unable to crack the ice and plunge toward some kind of deeper understanding, afraid to drown.

Given how the previous year had gone, it was a surprise when autumn and winter tottered along without serious incident. A movie I wrote opened and for one week it became the number #2 movie in the country and the #1 comedy. It was a very slow week.

We were cooking dinner one night when Susan said:

"I have something to tell you."

"Please tell me it's good."

"I think it's good."

"Okay, what?"

"I'm pregnant."

Staggered and thrilled, we embraced. Everything was going to be better. We would now finally put my mother's death, Bill's death, and the miscarriage behind us. We would honor the past and move bravely into the future. We dared imagine life would get a little easier. When we told my father, after offering his congratulations he informed us that he once again confronted his girlfriend about the phone calls and this time she came clean. So you're going to break up with her, I said. Because who would choose to remain with a woman who was so unstable she would telephone-harass his now pregnant daughter-in-law.

Someone who wanted to continue having sex with the woman.
He still refused to break up with her.

Indefatigable, indeed.

With the passage of time, it's harder to not be more understanding of Dad's predicament. He had lost his spouse, and in
his seventies the actuarial tables were not comforting.

Darkness was encroaching.

Who could blame him for howling like a wolf.

* * *

Tuesday afternoon less than a week after the appointment
with Dr. Moscowitz where he noticed suspicious activity up
and down the sides of my neck and Susan and I have gone out
to lunch. She has agreed to leave her office and meet me at a
Chinese restaurant so I'm not staring at the phone waiting for
it to ring. We talk about everything except the test results.
Since our family is expanding from three to four we wonder
whether we should we stay in the city. Perhaps move to the
country? Or California? Los Angeles played the part of a soul-
sucking void the first time I lived there, although my life was
different then.

So much to consider.

Without an appetite, I force myself to eat some pork lo
mein. After lunch Susan ditches work to accompany me home,
where there is a message on the answering machine from Dr.
Moscowitz. *On the answering machine!* A disembodied voice
tells me the result:

The test indicates lymphoma.

It's official.

In the lexicon of the comedy writers' room, here is the
quintessentially bad version.

We immediately get into a cab and shoot down to the doctor's office, again without an appointment. Arriving, we find it

packed with geriatrics, people meant to be there, benighted denizens of Medical World. They are old, decrepit. They know who Ava Gardner is and remember when the Lindbergh baby was kidnapped. What am *I* doing here?

The doctor's head nurse tells us to come back in an hour. We go for coffee and I'm careening between thinking about my funeral and vowing to treat the cancer like I'm Charles Bronson in *Death Wish* and it's the punks who killed my family (which, in a sense, it actually *is*). Buzzing with caffeine, we return to the doctor's office and are ushered in. The doctor is serene as a Japanese garden, easy for him. Susan is even-keeled. I thrum like a gong.

"You have a low-grade, follicular, mixed cell lymphoma," Dr. Moscowitz tells me in a smooth, don't-freak-out tone.

"What does that mean, low-grade?"

"It's indolent."

"Indolent?" I repeat. "Like it's lying in a hammock wearing a white suit and smoking a cigarette?" Susan puts her hand on my thigh. Steady, tiger. "Where is it?"

"It's presenting in Stage 4."

Those are the last two words anyone wants to hear. Like a friend that overshares, I knew them too well. Still, for some reason, I asked—

"What does *that* mean?"

"It's all over." My stomach drops four inches. All over. An unfortunate choice of words in so *many* ways. "The good news is that your organs are clear."

Breathe, breathe, breathe . . .

"And Stage 4 is—?"

"It's staged at 1 to 4."

"Four being the most critical." For some reason, I am trying to sound like a clinician. Why am I saying things we already know? The doctor remains silent. In this grim comedy, he is the straight man. "Is it curable?"

"It's treatable."

"Then what?"

"It tends to recur."

"On everyone?"

"Don't panic."

Who would panic? Doesn't everyone, upon learning they have cancer, a disease that could likely kill them, suddenly, through sheer force of will, lower their blood pressure and act like an old school nightclub crooner after his third whiskey, easy does it, cue the band, and swing? Why would anyone *panic*?

"But it's treatable?" In repetition there is comfort.

"Absolutely."

*Treatable* is vague in the extreme. "Treatable as in we treat it for a while and then you die? Or treatable as in you live a normal life span?"

"It means that we can treat it," he says, which does nothing to reassure me.

As we're leaving the office the doctor actually tells me to "smile." He wishes us well and tells us he's going to France for two weeks.

*I'm going to France.*

The words are innocent enough, they've been said before by many people. But this morning they stick in my craw.

*I have cancer, but you are going to France.*

*You* will be sipping Bordeaux. *I* will be sipping chemotherapy.

Why does this seem so profoundly *wrong*? Like the man from Riverside Memorial Chapel who told Dad he was sorry for the inconvenience.

And it's springtime. Central Park is in bloom. Susan is in bloom. All around me life is burgeoning.

\* \* \*

I have been thrust into a tangled netherworld.

A platitude: if you have to have cancer, lymphoma's the one. Lymphoma's the one! That's a laugh. It sounds like a campaign slogan, a bumper sticker. I've never even written the word before last week. All I know about lymphoma is that it can kill you.

*Lymphoma.*

What is a lymph anyway? Science was never my subject. The last science course I took was in high school. It was called Project Physics, and it was geared toward students for whom the grasping of actual physics was at best a faint hope. The beauty part—this being the early 1970s, the class was graded by self-evaluation. With the audacity of Hannibal leading the Carthaginian elephants over the mountains, I shamelessly gave myself an A. The teacher, who knew a fraud when he saw one, changed it to a C. If I had given myself a B he might have tolerated it, but an A he could not allow, never mind it was self-evaluation. And now, years later, *I* personally was a laboratory test the results of which would be considerably more important than a grade on my high school transcript.

The Merriam-Webster dictionary defines lymph as: *a pale coagulable fluid that bathes the tissues, passes into lymphatic channels and ducts, and is discharged into the blood by way of the thoracic duct.*

After learning this, I am still confused. Continuing my extensive research, it becomes clear the lymphatic system is a complex network of lymphoid organs. I also learn the lymphatic system is a major component of the immune system.

I had no idea.

The lymph system looks like a map of the New York City subways, with tracks going up and down Manhattan, into the Bronx of the head, veering off to the Queens and Brooklyn of the extremities. The analogy is inexact, but nonetheless conveys the idea of a complex, twenty-four hour a day transportation grid that carries lymph fluid rather than tired straphangers. Tonsils, those much-maligned pieces of seemingly randomly placed flesh located in the back of our necks, are part of the process. This is disappointing since mine were ripped from my throat when I was five years old as part of an epic removal of children's tonsils undertaken by the medical profession of that era in order to finance their new patios.

Lymphoma, then, is *a tumor of lymphoid tissue.* Apparently, I have cancer of something I didn't even know I had. For someone who prides himself on being well-informed it is disorienting to be blindsided. Like being hit with a tax bill for a property no one told me I owned, one with squatters that want to kill me.

And there is no way to appeal it.

Well, I think, they may *want* to kill me, these squatters, but *will* they?

The worst aspect of learning that your cancer is Stage 4 is the knowledge that that there is no Stage 5. But I am by nature an optimist and intend to find some ray of light. This proves exceedingly difficult. A little research reveals that the average survival rate for what I have is about six years. Six short years during which the shadow of early death is ever-present. Gone by forty-three, if I even live that long. Best-case scenario is remission, another recurrence, one more remission, and then—

Oh, fuck.

# PART 2
## SPRING CAN REALLY HANG YOU UP THE MOST

H ere's the truth: I am not one of those people who need a wake-up call to appreciate life. I chose to be a writer because it would afford me new experiences, allow me to continue to explore and absorb what is around me. No one would describe me as perfectly in tune with the world, but I have at least been trying to pay attention and have accrued a few benefits from that strategy.

Entire belief systems have been built on less than the glory of Central Park in the springtime. The light in Manhattan at dawn and at certain times in the late afternoon seems painted by Vermeer and I already *know* it. No one has to tell me. All right, that is not entirely true. Too often, I rush and there are plenty of times I pay no heed to that painterly Vermeer light slanting through the window because I'm waiting for a business call and—*Why hasn't that guy called, he said he was going to call today, is the project still happening?*—who has time for light appreciation when there are groceries to buy and a mortgage to be paid and the kitchen sink is leaking again, I thought the super fixed it. Allegra is dancing a toddler two-step but I'm distracted because the dishes need to be washed and didn't I just wash them yesterday and isn't it Susan's turn before I collapse with exhaustion in front of a television.

I perform tasks too quickly, am generally too impatient. Too, too, too.

But I'm an appreciator! I don't need lessons in gratitude! So many things in my life provide joy, yes, and I know it thank you very much! But this joy is like the blossom of a cactus flower which manifests gorgeously for a night before it mysteriously retreats and the spiny plant assumes its day-to-day character. It's exhausting to think this way. Draining. I want to go to sleep. As if I'll ever be relaxed enough to do that again.

So, I have cancer and I really *am* going to die. That's my first thought.

My second thought is death means Susan will be raising the kids alone, so guilt comes skidding to a halt, right on top of grief. Fiasco as a husband and father, AWOL from life, a paternal disaster in my own soon-to-be-dead eyes. My mother introduced me to art and books. Dad taught me how the world works. Will I leave no personal legacy for my kids? Allegra will barely remember me and the unborn one inside Susan whom we haven't even named yet will have no memories of me at all.

Here's the third thought: I arrive at the Pearly Gates—please excuse the convenient metaphor—and St. Peter, or Shlomo the Gate Attendant, or whoever the myth of your choice places there sees my name on his list of the recently deceased. And he looks up from his clipboard and says, What was your profession, sir? I tell him I was a writer. And he says, Have I heard of you?

The question every writer gets at parties: What have you done?

So.

My professional life in a nutshell circa 1993: a single movie credit, TV shows I wouldn't watch, plays performed at regional theatres, and a few one acts that were staged in New York. Through a variegated career in the entertainment business, it was easy to affect an attitude of slight remove because however slowly things might be progressing, as far as fulfilling my vast potential went, there was nothing but time. And now it appears the race could be over while I am still stumbling out of the starting blocks.

We leave the doctor's office and are walking toward the subway. People swirl around us on the street as if nothing is wrong. Don't they know the whole world is different now? That the Earth has tilted off its axis? Don't they know?

My obituary:

> **Seth Greenland, dead at 37**
> *Screenwriter-playwright Seth Greenland died yesterday. Along with the hip-hop classic* Who's the Man? *he wrote a lot of other stuff you've never heard of. His best-known play—and best known would be an exaggeration since it didn't exactly set the world on fire—was* Jungle Rot, *a comedy about the assassination of Patrice Lumumba, an African leader that no one who isn't a Marxist remembers. He worked on a sitcom starring Ricky Schroder, an act that he justified to himself by saying, Well, John Houseman worked on it, too, and* he worked with Orson Welles. *Prior to that, Greenland did time as a construction worker, lobster fisherman, and freelance journalist of no particular distinction. He was a graduate of Connecticut College and earned an MFA at NYU Film School which, if his credits are any indication, he did not put to good use. He is survived by his wife Susan, and two children. All of them deserved better. Funeral services will be someplace other than Riverside Memorial Chapel since they supervised the interment of his late mother and buried her facing the wrong direction.*

* * *

After receiving the diagnosis from my internist, along with his travel plans, a consideration of options occurs. Do I search high and low, scour every medical report and journal, talk to all the experts in the homeopathic, allopathic, Ayurvedic, Chinese, and folk medicine worlds?

I do not.

You hope to get through life without ever knowing the meaning of the word *oncologist*. Like numismatist, or philatelist, it is one of the words that flies through the ether, swirls around, and then usually sails off before landing anywhere nearby. And no one wants to say the words *My oncologist*. Here is a short list of phrases preferable to My oncologist:

My mounting debt

My persistent skin rash

My cellmate

Many people never have to say "My oncologist." Since my mother has recently died of cancer, not only is the locution familiar, I know an actual oncologist. His name is Dr. James Speyer, and despite his inability to keep my mother alive, something probably no one could have done, I like him. I accompanied my mother to several of her appointments, and he had visited her regularly when she was hospitalized so we had already shared a number of interactions. In his forties, tall, rail-thin, and possessed of a manner that suggests he is always and entirely in control, he exudes a dispassionate air appropriate to an occupation that calls for him to deal with people in extremis.

As Susan and I sit in Dr. Speyer's office which, like that of the peripatetic Dr. Moscowitz, is at NYU Medical Center, there is a conspicuous sense of déjà vu. It's eighteen months since my mother died, and now I am the chosen one, moved up from the undercard, here for the main event. Visiting a physician with a sick parent, although painful, is the correct order of things. The parent is significantly older, and is expected to precede you in death, usually by decades. But so little time has elapsed since I was last in this office that being there is disorienting. Why am I seated across from Dr. Speyer? Shouldn't we have been talking about my mother? Where has the veil gone, the one separating me from mortality? Everything is awry.

At least he doesn't act glad to see me.

After a quick exam, Dr. Speyer tells us I have inflamed nodes everywhere. Inflamed is a euphemism for cancerous and I appreciate his less invasive choice of adjective. As for the word *everywhere*, that is more problematic. It is akin to hearing the score of a football game is 49-0.

A comeback is improbable.

As I run my fingertips up and down my neck, the nodes feel like subcutaneous almonds. This, too, is how they feel in the area above my thighs. And, apparently, I have a couple of tumors in my abdomen the size of oranges. *Oranges!* While blindly living my life, rising, working, chasing Allegra around the apartment, going to the movies, shopping for dinner, eating, drinking, and sleeping, a cancerous army has infiltrated, caught me totally unawares, utterly routed my defenses. They have pulled off a Pearl Harbor attack and I am the Battleship Arizona, obliterated at anchor, sinking beneath the surface. And still, they are growing.

"Is it curable?" I ask. It's a question I will repeatedly be asking. It's the kind of question you ask until you hear the answer you want. If it's curable, then nothing else really matters. You can undergo any kind of treatment they devise, withstand whatever medieval abuse the medical profession invents as long as the end result is a cure. *Curable* trumps everything. *It's curable* beats your own island in Tahiti. It beats you've won the lottery. It beats anything since it means you can go back to believing you will have something approaching a normal life span.

"It's treatable," Dr. Speyer says.

"Treatable?" I ask. That word again. *Treatable.* Doctors love it. So equivocal.

"We can control it." *Well, that's good.* "But it tends to return." Didn't Dr. Moscowitz say that, too? Why can't they disagree on something?

"How often?"

"Usually."

"Then what happens?"

"We treat you again."

I nod, barely moving my chin. My breathing is shallow.

Susan pipes up: "What happens to the male reproductive ability with chemotherapy?"

I look at her. *What* did she just ask? This seems like a complete nonsequitur. We have a child and another is on the way. She might as well be wondering whether it will affect my ability to play the trombone.

"Why are you asking this? I say.

"I'm just curious."

Dr. Speyer stares at us impassively.

"Why are you worried about the integrity of my sperm cells?"

"I just am, okay?" Then she turns her attention back to Dr. Speyer. "So, what happens?"

"The reproductive ability can get scrambled," he says. I shake my head, mystified. What does this have to do with anything?

Chemotherapy starts the following week. I want to get going that afternoon. If they had told me to run to Philadelphia and back, swim the Hudson, wrestle an alligator—I would have done it. But they are making me wait. The first dose takes several hours and the next four an hour each. One week like this, then two weeks off, repeat the process for the next six months. I'm in a clinical trial, a therapy not yet approved for general use. I don't want what everyone else is getting. Give me the purest toxic cocktail imaginable. This Long Island Iced Tea of the lymphoma world will consist of cyclophosphamamide and fludarabine with a compazine chaser for the nausea.

Bottoms up!

We leave the office in what passes for a positive frame of mind. I am fighting the helplessness and despair that keep trying to infiltrate my barely maintained sense of calm. I have vowed to be relentlessly upbeat, since I know that if cracks begin to appear the edifice can quickly crumble. Susan is being strong and I am aware of how hard that must be. After all, she is pregnant. It is June now and she will deliver in November, assuming the pregnancy continues to go well. But how can we assume anything now? How can we know that one disaster will not follow another?

\* \* \*

In the spring of a recent year, Susan, Drew, and I were walking down West 79th Street in Manhattan, on our way to meet a friend for dinner. The architecture on the block between Columbus and Amsterdam Avenues has not changed, which lends it a timeless flavor, and I have walked down that bit of pavement in my twenties, thirties, forties, fifties, and now my early sixties. Whether it's because I was fortunate enough to be in good physical health with no aching joints or other crippling signs of aging, or because I had returned to the city in whose streets so much of my life has played out, or because the shifting shadows on the buildings at twilight create a subtly hypnotic effect, I felt myself for a moment become unstuck in time which is to say that it was briefly impossible to situate myself in a chronological place. The feeling only lasted for an instant but it was remarkably liberating. When I returned from my brief reverie to the present, I reflected on the difference between the ages one lives through and noticed that I was less eager to get to the restaurant where we were meeting our friend than I would have been years earlier, less eager to jump-start the evening, and increasingly keen to savor the moment in which we found ourselves. There's a physical slowing down that comes with age but also a development of the perception that allows a person to more easily occupy a single moment, to luxuriate in it, without rushing headlong to the next one.

There were several things that bothered me about being told definitively that I had cancer, the first one being that I had cancer. Then there was the seeming imminence of death which implied the life I had planned was not going to happen.

It is slightly disconcerting to report at this quarter century distance that what bothered me the most about the situation was that I would not get to live out the creative dreams I believed that I had been put on this planet to fulfill. Yes, my children might be fatherless but if I was the kind of undependable failure who died from cancer in his thirties then it would be better for them in the long run. And my wife would realize she had married someone whose destiny turned out to be that of a victim. The opportunity to further impress my father would be lost because I would expire in media res.

When I recall the hollowness of my reaction upon hearing the news, it brings me up short. Back then, I thought any idiot can get married and have a family. The list of idiots who have done that would stretch from here to the outer reaches of the solar system. But to be an artist took talent! We're *special*. In case you missed it, the italicization of the word special is meant to convey irony. It's hard to believe that the prospect of death obliterating my inconsequential career was my deepest concern. But then I wonder, was that actually how I reacted or am I remembering it incorrectly? Everything was so greased with fear that it's hard to recollect the details with clarity. But I know this: from the time I first heard the snare thwack and the womp of the bass drum that kicked off "Like a Rolling Stone,"

I fantasized about being an artist of some kind. Before I could articulate it, before I could conceive it in lucid terms; whatever that ineffable feeling conjured by Bob Dylan was, I needed more. Because my public school did not offer guitar, I took up the trumpet only to discover that I was unburdened by talent. Art class: not Picasso. But my ability to write showed up at an early age and by this point I was a decade in as a professional. Almost everything up until the diagnosis was throat clearing, breathing exercises, singing scales. The idea that I would be cut down before I got a chance to belt would be the perfect tragic ending to what had become a comic life. How could I impress my father if I were dead?

Perhaps Dad's literary aspirations were what gave me the idea. His own background might have inspired him to write like Henry Roth or Abraham Cahan, chroniclers of the New York tenement streets, whose books are on the shelf to my right. After my rogue grandfather flew the coop my father grew up with his mother, younger sister, and older brother in a two-room, ground floor apartment in the 1920s South Bronx. My grandmother worked as a beautician and attended to clients in the front room. As a kid, my father would go down to the flower district before dawn, buy carnations, and sell them to swains at Yankee Stadium. He never enrolled full-time in college although he made a point of telling me he took courses at the New School. Later, he developed into a serious reader and was conversant in subjects like history, economics, art, politics, and how to tie a Windsor knot. In 1942 he joined the Army to get away from his father, for whom he worked in an auction gallery, and who occupied a higher economic class than the family he deserted. After the war, following stints as an aspiring theatrical producer and a press agent, he found his way to the advertising business and there he thrived, eventually founding his own agency in 1958 that he operated until 1993, winning awards, recognition, and large servings of self-esteem.

His picture was in newspapers and magazines. He was occasionally on television. There's a framed photograph of him in my foyer standing with Ed Koch and Andy Warhol. He made it to the top. The skiing, tennis, and horseback riding in Van Cortlandt Park a manifesto from a young man whose mother didn't have the money to pay the rabbi to perform a bar mitzvah. Like President Reagan, also from modest circumstances, he behaved as if he had been born waving his hat astride a rearing steed.

He hit me when I was a kid. That sounds more dramatic than it was. It didn't happen a lot, and never with an object, but I was spanked, 1960s-style like so many of my boomer cohort. His temper would seethe and blow, then I'd get bent over and have my backside swatted. My less confrontational sibling rarely stuck his head over the parapet. But I could not keep my mouth shut and Dad was not able to brook my lip. The final episode occurred when I was thirteen. Imagine the living room of our house on Brite Avenue, a big old suburban mock-Tudor pile with a basement and an attic. Rows of windows on three sides, the leafy street to my left, backyard to my right, and sunlight pouring in. I mouthed off about who remembers what and he slapped me across the face so hard the blow sent my horn-rimmed glasses flying across the room. I was stunned, but stoic. My nonreaction must have been a valve for his wrath because the hostile energy crackling between us immediately dissipated. The commotion seemed ridiculous. That was the only time he ever hit me in the face and he never struck me again. Left in the dust by my Bronx playboy grandfather, alternately furious and remorseful, my father had responsibilities. He was making a payroll with sixty people on it. They didn't talk back. He didn't know how to handle his mouthy son and did not possess either the vocabulary or the inclination to peacefully unpack conflict.

Those who come up from under who are not professional comedians are rarely self-deprecating and Dad was no exception. He was serious and literal, dark suits and gray fedoras. There is a stereotype of Jewish husbands of his generation being henpecked and when I became aware of it I was shocked. Dad was about as henpecked as Henry VIII. Perhaps it was because he was ten years older than my mother, but theirs was a marriage cast in the traditional mold, which is to say she worked for him. Not technically, but our life was set up to serve the needs of the provider. My mother quit working— she had been a department store buyer—when they got married and devoted herself to running the house and looking good for her husband. And she did look good. Svelte and stylish with impeccable taste, she was a Bensonhurst duchess, and viewed Drew and me as extensions of her, which caused problems. More than anything, she wanted to please our father. This was a quality I picked up. It didn't run my life; it was never the melody, but it was always the bass.

When I announced I was going to film school, Dad was all for it, like he had never heard the word lawyer. And now the palimpsest of his memory, the jostling suburban husband and father of young children, the equanimous old man ambling on a Florida beach, his enterprising boyhood in the shadow of the Grand Concourse, is threaded with all the layered scenes of my different lives as I amble down West 79th Street in the early evening.

\* \* \*

After Dr. Speyer confirms the news, Dad arrives for dinner. He is taking time away from his insatiable Brazilian girlfriend whose husband died of AIDS, something that still does not bother him despite my repeatedly pointing it out. Although he is clearly enjoying what he views as his spectacular good fortune at having copious amounts of geriatric sex with a woman half his age, she is tightly wound which is a polite way of saying probably bipolar and he needs a break from their mercurial trysts.

I pour him two fingers of scotch over ice and we sit in the tropically-hued living room. He leans back and takes in the sight of his sick son, the two of us doing a passable impression of holding it together. His wife is gone and now *this*. I am everyone's new problem. Susan's parents have just buried an adult child. Is my father wondering if this is to be his fate?

Dad offers encouragement and support, and while his words are comforting, what is more meaningful is his presence because I have learned there are no words that can make any of this better. I'm experiencing an impending sense of deep isolation, of remove, of being nudged away from everything familiar and comforting, from family and work and friends, perhaps most of all from love, and wanting to desperately cling to all of it as it slips from my grasp, and words won't change any of that. It isn't that love is being denied; quite the opposite. But it is the anticipation of love's absence that awaits in the cold and dark of wherever I'm sliding. The utter aloneness. And all of this is impossible for me to verbalize.

After a few minutes of forced good cheer, unable to think of anything more to jabber about, I pick up that day's *New York Times* from the coffee table.

My father asks what I'm reading.

"The obituaries," I tell him. "The sports page for the terminally morbid."

"I check them every morning to make sure I'm still alive," he says.

Susan makes leek soup for dinner. Dad has been eating healthily for years, no butter, lots of fish, vegetables to beat the band. Leek soup thrills him.

"I did an Internet search on lymphoma," Susan says. "There's a specialist in Berlin doing a clinical trial that sounds promising. I made a phone call and—"

I cut her off: "Let's talk about something else." Taking the sting out with a smile.

"Some of that stuff is pretty weird," Dad says. "People getting lambs' glands shot into their rumps."

Wanting to change the subject to something more cheerful I ask: "What do you think happens when we die?"

Dad and Susan look at each other. In a shared instant, they decide to humor me. "Maybe it's like in *Carousel*," Susan says. Before she became an attorney, she was a theatre major.

"The musical?" From my father.

We have recently seen a production of *Carousel*. It's all about death. At the time I experienced it as a pleasurable couple of hours with some great songs.

"The Starkeeper lets you look down on Earth," Susan says.

"So, the Christians and the Buddhists missed it," I say. "But Rodgers and Hammerstein got it right?"

"You're not dying," Dad says. He eats another spoonful of soup. The room is quiet. My father asks Susan if she has used butter in the soup.

"No butter," she assures him.

"Low fat," he says. "I like that."

"Sure, low fat," I say to my father. "Live to a hundred." It's meant as a joke, but it comes out with a bitter aftertaste. He nods. Susan tries to smile, then looks away.

"I'm going through your mother's things," Dad says, "to give them away. I could use a hand." This is the last thing I want to do. I tell him I would be happy to help.

That night we are in our bedroom. I am seated on the bed and Susan stands, looking out the window. She is weeping because, unwilling to articulate it for obvious reasons, she knows there is a distinct chance that relatively soon I am going to not be here. Sympathy would be the right move for me, the smart and sensitive gesture, to hold and comfort her in this time of distress. But since *I* am the one who is ill that is difficult. Can I put her needs before mine at this moment; be the rock that she requires?

I would like to be that rock but right now my heart is not in it. I am reeling, my conception of life shattered.

And I am too busy feeling sorry for myself.

When we decided to get married it was assumed we would spend the rest of our lives together. When you are in your thirties and hear the words *the rest of our lives* it is natural to believe that will be a long time. We have been married for less than four years. This brings up the question of longevity. Doesn't the *Bible* routinely refer to the human life span as "three score and ten"? I always thought that was one of the few instances where the *Bible* might be accurate. By my calculation, whoever wrote that section might have been off by at least a score and a half. And what of my own family? My grandfathers, men who ate Eastern European cooking (the culinary equivalent of arterial sclerosis) their entire lives, who considered pinochle exercise, who smoked and drank with abandon, both lived past seventy. Dad has already made it past seventy and is going strong.

I am relatively young and vigorous. Then what has caused my cells to behave like British soccer hooligans on a beach weekend in Spain? What has caused my cancer? The toxic environment that swirls around us? Chemicals in water? Additives in food? I went to summer camp in the mountains and every few weeks trucks would ride through spraying DDT, enveloping all of Camp Mah-Kee-Nac in a toxic fog. The gestation period of certain cancers can last decades. Had mine originated in the innocence of a long-ago summer, a time of baseball, fireflies, and incipiently mutating cells?

Or perhaps it is just incredibly rotten luck.

As Susan tries to drift off, I think about the music I want played at my funeral. "Who Knows Where the Time Goes" by the English folk singer Sandy Denny is one of my favorite songs. An achingly beautiful meditation on loss and the passage of time and as much as I love it—a little on the head. A friend of ours had attended a funeral where they played "Sing, Sing, Sing," by Benny Goodman, a raucous swing tune. A bold choice but it wouldn't work for me. If "Who Knows Where the Time Goes" is too elegiac, "Sing, Sing, Sing" was too comical. It's fine to tell funny stories, but a comedy soundtrack seems tone deaf. How to strike a balance between sobriety and mischief, the twin poles by which I've been navigating my entire life. Charles Mingus's powerful tribute to Lester Young, "Goodbye, Porkpie Hat," could work but while its smoky Kool menthol tones would create a nightclub feeling that certain mourners might appreciate, Charles Mingus wrote it for someone else and it strikes me as presumptuous, not to say unoriginal, for it to be played at my funeral.

I put a pin in the music and try and think about the readings. An elegy by Shelley? Too pretentious. "Funeral Blues" by Auden? An astonishingly good poem but where is the intersection of Auden and me other than we both write in the same language? Something American, by Whitman, perhaps "O Captain, My Captain"? While the merit of the poem is unchallenged, a mourner declaiming it at my funeral would feel like an overdramatic moment from a high school play. And I imagine the friend I ask to read it reporting, Seth wanted me to read "O Captain, My Captain," and rolling his eyes.

Susan's eyes are closed. She is oblivious to my ruminations. Is she asleep?

Quietly, I say, "I want a bagpipe player."

"Where?"

"At my funeral."

Bagpipes are a bold stroke. No one is singing so there will be an absence of lyrics to parse, the sound is sorrowful, and a lone piper strikes an indelible image. There's no Scottish in me but Susan's family name is MacLeod and it is our daughter's middle name. I am Scots-adjacent, good enough.

Pleased with myself, I say, "Should he be in a kilt or would the kilt be too much?"

"You're not being funny."

"I want a guy from one of those British Army outfits. The Royal Scots Fusiliers."

"Shut up, please."

"What's with you?"

"Stop joking around. I don't like it."

"How do you think "My Way" would sound on the bagpipes?" I continue, unable to stop beating this baleful fancy to an unsightly pulp. "He could do a whole Sinatra medley. Then I want the pallbearers in sharkskin suits and porkpie hats. I was just now thinking about Lester Young who not only pretty much invented the jazz saxophone but was also famous for wearing a porkpie hat," I nonsensically tell my wife, who has other things to worry about, like being married to a lunatic. Unable to stop, I tell her, "I want six guys who look like Lester Young to empty a pint of Hennessy on my grave."

Susan props herself on her elbow and looks at me. She is not pleased. The gallows humor is a good coping tool for some, less so for others. It's hard to stop the logorrheic schtick but I get the message. Kissing her goodnight, I try to think simple thoughts, easy thoughts, springtime, and flowers (*Should* I be involved in choosing the ones for my funeral?), and the long-ago trip to Egypt which gets me ruminating about—why is it so hard to stay in the illuminated area, the safe area?—olden times. When the ancients heard thunder, what was the explanation? They thought that someone they could not see, someone who probably lived in the sky, was mad at them.

Super mad. So mad, in fact, that he was unleashing a barrage of very loud noise and bright lights to scare the shit out of them. How could they propitiate this angry entity? They decided to beg him to stop.

Really beg.

Together.

In a group.

And then have a bake sale.

Thus, religion was born.

Clearly, this is an opportunity for some roots exploration.

I glance over at Susan who is now sleeping peacefully. At least she appears to be sleeping peacefully. Maybe she's only faking since she knows if I think she's asleep that will be the end of my melancholy rambling.

Half an hour crawls past. I climb out of bed and sit at my desk. My home office in our apartment has a window, a detail I mention to distinguish it from an actual closet. It is a closet off the bedroom fourteen floors above West 76th Street—you might say it looms over the funeral home—and I sit at the desk gazing out the window. To distract myself from thoughts of death I make a mental list of musicians I've seen perform live: Led Zeppelin at the Fillmore East in what was their first American gig, Dexter Gordon at the Village Vanguard, the Rolling Stones at Madison Square Garden, which gets me thinking about Brian Jones, dead in a swimming pool, and this leads to me to ponder all the musicians who died young: Eric Dolphy, dead at thirty-six, Charlie Parker, dead at thirty-six, Clifford Brown, dead at twenty-six, Charlie Christian, dead at twenty-two. And that's only a fraction of the jazz world. In rock there is the whole Buddy-Jimi-Janis-there's-a-new-one-every-week tradition. I am ripe. Obscure, but ripe. And compared to some of the dead musicians, I'm *old*.

In thinking about all the dead young musicians it strikes me that remarkably few of them died of cancer. I don't envy them because *they're dead*, but at least most of them avoided chemotherapy. While the medical community has devised countless new treatments, and continues to work assiduously on the problem, there is still no reliable cure for cancer. There are, however, lots of lapel ribbons in exciting new colors. There's peach for Endometrial, orchid for Testicular, and periwinkle for Esophageal. Since when is periwinkle even a color? It sounds like the name of a fairy in an obscure 17th century English poem written by Andrew Marvell. The lapel ribbons represent a bargain between the wearer and the deity of their choice: in exchange for not burdening them with a horrifying disease, they will wear this colorful ribbon. The ribbons are essentially narcissistic.

There is an upside to cancer: it's a chance to display courage. I wasn't born poor or disfigured. I never went hungry unless you count fasting on Yom Kippur and then I usually cheated. I didn't have to serve in Vietnam. This will be a chance to prove my mettle, show my spine. Cancer will be my Battle of Iwo Jima, my Khe Sanh, and judging by the choice of metaphor my license to be overly dramatic. I will be strong, inspirational. I know how to suffer, after all. I've seen it at the movies. Read about it. I've been a lifelong New York Knicks fan.

Suffering has a venerable pedigree. Who can forget Tiny Tim, or that girl in *Love Story*? Not to mention King Lear, Madame Bovary, and late-career Elvis. Western culture is addicted to suffering, as long as it's not our own. And why is this?

Because we believe it to be ennobling.

Some cancers are deadlier than others, and while it isn't necessarily the death sentence it was perceived to be as recently as thirty years ago, it still isn't what you want to hear your doctor tell you. What you want to hear your doctor say is, You're fine. See you next year. Or, failing that, Have you considered switching to margarine? You don't want to hear *cancer*. If you're anything like I am, you don't even want to hear "cancer" in casual conversation because the associations that spring to mind are so unpleasant.

Cancer's not *sexy*. It's quite un-sexy, actually. It's the complete and total opposite of sexy if you want to know the truth. In a society as shallow, youth-driven, and generally cretinous as ours, cancer is everything you're supposed to not want. In the Misfortune Sweepstakes, people prefer to win diabetes, or Crohn's Disease, or lupus. Whether or not this (admittedly anecdotal) preference is based on anything other than perception is an entirely different question. It remains that cancer is the boogeyman of words, the one most guaranteed to knife the fearful hearts of the largest number of people.

Words are like bread for me. This is one of the reasons I have always been a great reader. Perhaps *great* is an exaggeration. What I am is someone who reads a lot; magazines, newspapers, the ingredients on food packages. Books, too, obviously. When confronted with something new, my first reaction is to read about it. My means of bringing what little order I can to the maelstrom that is a Day in the Life of Me is the accrual of knowledge.

Crawling back to bed in the middle of the night, I assure myself there will be consolation in at least knowing a few helpful things.

The next morning is like reopening a wound. We return to the Barnes and Noble on Broadway and 83rd Street for some intensive shopping. So great is my agitation I barely remember having walked there when we arrive. We could have gone to the library but I want to own these books I was after, to absorb their contents, truly *possess* them. I fill my arms with what I hope will be inspirational paperbacks that have sold millions of copies, bringing succor to an international community of the afflicted. At home I devour the books as if the information in their pages is an elixir in itself.

I read and read.

But the reading is not providing the hoped-for comfort and rather than relaxing and going to sleep, the bats in my skull pinwheel in crazy flight. The narrative in which I find myself is the kind I avoid; one where the antagonist is faceless, implacable, relentless.

Additional books are bought. The pile swells. More reading, searching, examining, parsing, and wishing. But these books contain no answers I need; nor are they particularly inspiring. And not only aren't these books inspiring, they're boring. I hate most of them. One of them, by a doctor, I loathe with a particular intensity since it is his theory that anyone with cancer has caused it to occur. Themselves! As if a person who has just been diagnosed with cancer doesn't already have enough to feel shitty about. This is odious on so many levels it's hard to know where to start but I would like to begin by smacking this man on the bridge of his nose with a hardback copy of his execrable book, all the more galling for being a bestseller. What makes this doctor's malign theory so maddening is that by claiming a person has caused their own cancer it imbues that individual with an entirely false sense of control suggesting as it does that if they caused this mess, they can fix it, entirely eliding the random, out-of-control property of the disease with which it is much harder to make peace.

It is a guilty feeling hating these books because they are so well-meaning and I'm sure the authors are lovely people who are nice to their families, give generously to charity, and have a song in their hearts. Or not. Who cares? They are just so *earnest*. The only earnest I like is the one that completes the following title: *The Importance of Being—*. Otherwise, earnest is tiresome, dull, and, well, *earnest*.

There is nothing to help me to cope with this new reality that is going to ennoble me and then kill me, nothing to give hope that doesn't feel like recycled bromides, tired homilies for a quaking congregation. One of the books is written by a well-known magazine editor who had contracted a horrific and incurable disease the symptoms of which involved something going spectacularly wrong with his joints. In response, he screened videotapes of old comedies and claims to have laughed himself back to health in the flickering image of Groucho Marx. Good for him. The funny thing is that he was a rather serious man in his life. I, on the other hand, always viewed laughter as salutary and have been engaging in it regularly until my diagnosis, at which point, I stopped for a few days. No, I laughed my way *to* cancer. And now I'm supposed to laugh even more? It is counterintuitive. Groucho Marx will not work for me.

In the book by the laughing magazine editor, I learn that the physicist Linus Pauling claimed to have cured himself of cancer by using massive doses of vitamin C. Although Linus Pauling was possessed of a more capacious intelligence than I, this is clearly silly. I could take all the vitamin C in the world and still have cancer. Don't ask me how I know. I just do. Perhaps it is because no one else has ever replicated that result. There can be no medical cohort that could include only Linus Pauling and me.

I am bereft.

Where is the first-person account, written in a loose, amusing yet informative style by someone who has been through this terrifying experience and (big caveat) lived to write about it? How am I supposed to cope without a book? There is no other way for me to frame my story. I vow to write that book if I survive.

*   *   *

At least there is now a definitive plan of action. I'm going to have chemotherapy to make my body well (after destroying it). But what about the rest of me? What of the part that worries and wishes and envies and aspires and taps his fingers impatiently on the table? What of that part? And to whom can I talk about it? No one, because I'm too ashamed.

The heart of my childhood passed more than five decades ago and yet there are moments I remember with the vividness of a movie I saw last night; actors, setting, costumes. As a kid I wore dungarees and sometimes the zipper jammed. One afternoon at the house of a friend who lived down the street, I slipped into the bathroom just off the kitchen. A gang of kids played outside, their eager shouts still audible as I locked the door behind me. Nine years old and confident, I wanted to get back to the games as fast as possible. But I really had to take a leak. I unzipped the—wait—I didn't unzip anything. The zipper refused to go south. Increasingly determined, I struggled with my recalcitrant fly, but no luck. The physical pressure intensified. I *really* had to piss. The cries of my friends—*Car, car, C-A-R, stick your head in a pickle jar*—boomed in the street. Once more I tugged and nothing. Mounting panic as my muscles began to surrender. Before I was able to yank my belt over my hips and free the penis from its Fruit of the Loom prison my bladder emptied, leaving an accusatory stain on my pants that reported at top volume the disaster that had just occurred.

Little children wet their pants, a poised nine-year-old did not. In the bleak tradition of childhood, I would be mocked, labeled a "baby," made to feel that I possessed a deep and abiding flaw unique to me. I would be isolated (however briefly), eroded, and worst, recategorized. My "confidence," clearly fake, evaporated in the face of this potential humiliation. I was *fearful* of judgement and *shamed* by my predicament. At that moment I could have curled up in a thimble. My friend in whose bathroom I was suffering had recently managed to catch the skin of his actual penis in the zipper of his fly, but his mother and I were the only ones to witness that piece of egregious luck, and neither of us chose to add to his already considerable misery by mocking the predicament. It was cold comfort since I was alone with soaked blue jeans. I can still smell the reek of urine on the bathroom floor. That I was probably overdramatizing the entire event did not occur to me at the time. Until years later, I did not understand that no one is thinking about me because they're caught up in their own subjectivity. As a teenager, I walked stoned on cheap Mexican weed into a brightly lit fast food restaurant convinced every patron was staring at me. They were not. To this day I've yet to come up with an explanation more illustrative of how the world views us.

I made it to my bicycle, conveniently parked in the back of the house, and my friends were too distracted by the game they were playing to pay much attention when I pedaled down the driveway and yelled something about having to be home immediately, accompanying this announcement with a cheerful wave, before disappearing moistly into the distance.

If hope is "the thing with feathers," fear and its cousin shame are the snaky thing with scales. Their insidious, slithering movement and poisonous bite mark them as unwelcome intruders in the orchard of one's psyche. And yet they thrive. Much of human behavior can be understood through the twin prisms of fear and shame. This remains true even in our increasingly shameless era. We are fearful creatures by nature, even the chest-thumpers who have come to define a certain kind of American maleness. The proliferation of firearms can largely be attributed to fear; of crime, of difference, of reality. We're scared of failure, of losing what we have, of intimacy, of being judged, of aging. We're scared of death, which is one of the reasons it's become so antiseptic. Death happens out of sight. We don't even like to say "dead." Uncle Fred "passed away" or "passed on" or just "passed." Words designed to be whispered.

When I first started trying to write about cancer, it did not occur to me to explore the shame that arrived with the diagnosis because (a) it felt too personal and (b) I was *ashamed* that I had been ashamed (shame has infinite layers). But now it seems obvious that shame was a key component of the experience. It was imperative that no one who was not a close friend or family member be aware of what I was going through. It was bad enough that my wife had to know. How was I to project virility when my body was in crisis? What would this do to our sex life, already a dodgy proposition what with a baby on the way and the proclivity of the two-year-old with whom we were living to launch into leather-lunged arias the moment the lights went out?

I was terrified that people in Hollywood would find out and no one would hire me. One of the many Rules of Show Business is that employers hire who they want to hang out with. Who wants to hang out with cancer? Like failure, it is assumed you can catch it. (No one believes this on a conscious level. But the subliminal message is unmistakable.) In 1993, it was the moral equivalent of plague.

The movies are about illusion. There is no greater illusion than the belief that we are not going to die. Illness forces people to notice the man behind the curtain, the one gesturing them toward the shadows, the one they can ignore on the sunny days that, for a healthy person, are Monday through Sunday every week.

Understandably, Dad has none of this in mind. In an attempt to manage his own anxiety caused by having a son that might predecease him, he managed to spill the beans about what was going on to his friend Irwin. Irwin's son Donald, whom I barely knew, had just become engaged to a young woman I had never met. Coincidentally, this woman worked for the big Hollywood agency that represented me. Because I was so concerned that news of my condition would leak out and destroy my career—clear thinking was on hiatus; was the agency going to circulate a memo?—I called Donald's poor unsuspecting fiancée, who likely did not know I existed until someone passed her the receiver that day, and with a voice full of passion and fear, a voice that, frankly, must have sounded slightly unhinged, I implored her to keep news of my diagnosis secret. She was gracious and the conversation mercifully brief. To this day I have yet to meet her but if I did, my first order of business would be to apologize for that bonkers phone call.

Cancer allowed me to experience fear and shame simultaneously. The two gifts I least wanted were barreling down on me with the velocity and heft of a meteor. The fear, obviously, was of suffering and early death. But the feeling of shame was more complex. There is a cornucopia of reasons an American male abhors being perceived as weak. Evolution is a good place to begin. For all of our apps, advances in artificial intelligence, and impressive new strand-by-strand hair replacement techniques, we still possess the DNA of hunter/gatherers and even to those of us who have evolved to the point where we pay the bills by writing screenplays the idea of earning a paycheck is a lineal descendant of hurling a spear at a saber-tooth tiger. It isn't news to observe that males of my generation, raised by hard-ass fathers that had served in World War II, were expected to be strong and stoic. Some of us avoided this pathology, but the rest mostly "drank the Kool-Aid." And if we didn't actually *drink* it, we at least internalized the lesson. In a capitalist economy, weakness suggests penury. As a young husband and father with one child keeping me awake and another warming up in the wings, the idea that I might simultaneously fail in multiple roles because of *weakness* was a catastrophe around which I could barely wrap my mind. Never did I present myself as the hammer of Thor, but my self-image was one of strength, wholeness, and robust health. To discover that my system had betrayed me felt like losing control of my bladder when I was nine years old and urinating all over myself.

* * *

Birds wheel over the East River as a tanker makes its way south toward the Atlantic Ocean. It is a perfect day for a ramble in Central Park. Then what are Susan and I doing angling toward Memorial Sloan Kettering this Tuesday morning so soon after my diagnosis? Oncologists have subcategories, which was not something I knew when I began this odyssey. There is the breast cancer tribe, bone cancer specialists, doctors whose expertise is in cancers of the blood. After extensive research, we learn that the Lymphoma King in New York is Dr. Strauss at Memorial Sloan Kettering. I do not like the idea of going to Memorial Sloan Kettering for one reason. It's a *cancer* hospital. After reading the previous sentence, perhaps you're thinking: wait, you *have* cancer. Yes, I know. But it's not like I need to be reminded. I am aware this is childish, but I cling to my former existence, the one in which there is no illness.

Why are we going to see Dr. Straus? In hopes of getting that phone call from the governor intended to forestall a death row inmate's execution known as a second opinion, one that diverges from the first. Give me the familiar confines of NYU Medical Center, please.

This is a delicate distinction I am making, indicative of my delicate psychological state.

Here is the difference between the hospitals: when I go to NYU Medical Center, the patients I observe are there for orthopedic reasons, neonatal reasons, psychiatric reasons. I am one of many, a drop in a variegated sea, not singled out by my current, unenviable role. But at Memorial Sloan Kettering I will not be subsumed by that medical melting pot. Here, we all share the same affliction. Perhaps not the same variety (cancer

being a many-splendored thing), but we are partners in a particular kind of fretfulness. If this goes bad, it could go *really*
bad. To me, hearing the words *He's being treated at Sloan
Kettering* has an unmistakable whiff of doom. As far as I am
concerned they may as well have the words *Arbeit Macht Frei*
carved above the entrance since you were about as likely to get
out of this particular place alive as you were the concentration
camp where the phrase was first displayed. But my rational
mind knows this is a misapprehension—they've saved the lives
of countless people!—and I have forced a change in my own
thinking. The doctors here are cutting edge, doing things no
one else is doing. I tell myself to overcome my illogical feelings
and get on with it. I stare up at the building, red brick, stolid.
I do not want to go in.

Susan senses my uncertainty and tugs my arm. The appointment must be kept.

We enter the lobby and look around. It certainly seems like
a regular hospital. Patients in various states of torment, some
of it hidden, some not so hidden, can be seen asking questions
at the reception desk, waiting for the elevator, leaving the
building (they're leaving and they're still alive!).

But no one is here to have a baby. Susan will be having one
in a few months (let's not forget), just not in this place.

We ride the elevator surrounded by people dealing with
cancer. Either they've got it or someone close to them does. We
walk down the hushed hallway toward the doctor's office and
I glance into the sterile rooms; everyone's being treated for
cancer. Despite the antiseptic smell, the place is malodorous
with dismay. In every room, behind every desk, in every
patient's file which grows and grows, are malignancies as far as
the eye can see. The walls, the floors, the ceilings have all
absorbed the cancer gestalt, which, to my perfervid mind, feels
overwhelming. The building itself feels to me like it has cancer.

Are people cured in this place? I hope so, but why do I even think about that since I've been told there is no cure for lymphoma? Then why am I even here? Because second opinions are holy writ. Anyone who receives alarming medical news will recognize these words: *Did you get a second opinion?* It is a question that gets asked ad infinitum by one's friends in the usually vain hope that the doctor who made the initial diagnosis somehow screwed it up. That this does happen occasionally renders the question a good one. On the off chance that the inflamed lymph nodes and the tropical fruit-sized tumors were caused by something more benign, here we are, hoping wildly against hope that a medical professional will tell us this is all a big mistake.

In the waiting room tattered magazines beckon, a distraction, but who can even concentrate enough to read what's on their covers, so irrelevant are they, so unimportant and beside the point. Susan pretends to read a magazine. I chew my lip. Finally, we are given clearance to enter Dr. Strauss's unassuming office. The doctor is not there. In a chair, I try to fend off a panic attack. Before its onset, I am summoned into an exam room by a friendly, young Italian doctor who is doing his residency. We spent our honeymoon in Italy on the Amalfi coast only three years earlier and this resident's musical accent brings memories rushing back— lunch in Positano, a day trip to Capri, looking for Gore Vidal's house in Ravello (we didn't *know* him. We had just heard he owned a magnificent house), sunny, wine-fueled afternoons, and a boundless future. But now I leave Susan in Dr. Strauss's empty office. The Italian doctor examines me then takes all the slides and charts I've brought from NYU and distributes them to the various local panjandrums so they can weigh in. An RN with a brisk manner comes in and delivers a lecture about lymphoma, everything I already know. The experience is starting to assume a Kabuki aura, as if we are enacting roles; I am the patient, she is the caregiver, and it is our 137th performance, a half-filled Wednesday matinee. Someone opens a candy wrapper in the third row, and I try to stay focused on the actress with whom I am doing the scene.

Finally, Dr. Strauss arrives. Susan joins us. We had been warned that he was a tough guy but he turns out to be relatively benign, as it were. He examines me and says the tumors don't feel that big. I like him instantly. In my current state, I am a dog. If you scratch my head I will lick your hand. Immediately the whole day feels more worthwhile. My tail starts to wag.

He invites us into his office where he says, "You have a really crummy thing."

Thank you, Dr. Strauss. That is why I am here at the most famous cancer hospital in the world, just so you can tell me I have a crummy thing.

Then he tells me more crummy things I already know about low-grade, follicular mixed cell lymphoma. At this point I can teach a course in the subject. He is familiar with all the clinical trials we mention as befits his status as the Lymphoma King. He suggests that once complete remission is achieved (I love his optimism!) we should extract bone marrow and store it. In the event of a recurrence—*It tends to recur*—I could then have what is known as an "autologous" transplant, a transplant with one's own bone marrow. I do not want to do this, but I say I will consider it. It troubles me that I know what autologous means.

"So, Dr. Strauss," I say. "Is this curable?"

"There are a lot of misconceptions about lymphoma," he says. "And one of them is that it's incurable." Did I hear his correctly? This is not what Dr. Moscowitz said. This is not what Dr. Speyer said. *This* is sweeter than pie. If there is one reason for me to withstand the emotional workout a visit to

Memorial Sloan Kettering entails, it is to hear those words uttered by the Lymphoma King. But then he says, "We can't cure it yet—" And I deflate. *Yet?*

"Any idea of the timing?" Trying to keep the desperation out of my voice.

"Well," he says, expansively, "there are a lot of clinical trials going on. They're doing one at Stanford that looks particularly promising. It's a vaccine."

"Can that help me?"

"Not now."

Oh, I get it. It's incurable *now* but eventually, maybe not. Dr. Strauss's expertise does not extend to verb tenses. Apparently, it *will be* curable. If I can manage to survive for the twenty or so years it will take for this serum to be perfected, I should be fine. *That's* encouraging. We shake hands and he wishes us good luck. At least he's not going to France.

\* \* \*

Exhausted from the day, the emotional turbulence, the entire disrupted narrative—*I had a consultation at Memorial Sloan Kettering? And it was a second opinion because someone needed to hear he has cancer TWICE?!*—I stare at my record collection. It is nearly midnight and Susan is asleep because despite all the recent drama she still has to go to work every day. For all of my brio when in the company of mental health professionals, the state of relaxation that leads to sleep continues to elude me and I have an aversion to pills. Hundreds of albums rest on a living room shelf. I have been a record collector since I was ten. Now I finger the cardboard jackets, many still in their cellophane wrappers, slit open to allow removal and return of the discs and preserve the integrity of the object, a fetish for true music lovers; albums by Elvis Costello, the Ramones, Neil Young, the Allman Brothers,

Louis Armstrong, the Clash. Their presence, and all the associations they evoke—playing in a band as a kid, dancing, parties—are like the smell of dinner cooking. But it is to the blues section that my attention drifts and I pull out records by Otis Spann, Mississippi Fred MacDowell, and Freddie King, plangent sounds I've been listening to since high school. I put on an Otis Spann album I bought forever ago called *Walkin' The Blues*. The song *Going Down Slow* begins to play. I collapse on the couch and listen to Spann's deft left hand, his primal croak, waiting for them to palliate reality.

Reeling back to my adolescence, pushed by Otis Spann, I pull out my high school yearbook and open it to the senior section. The yearbook is clean as new snow on a winter morning. No one has written in it because I wanted—what did I want at the time?—a spotless document of a fraught period, one of insomnia, disappointment, and mild depression enlivened by the occasional rock concert, basketball game, or nocturnal emission. Ah, high school! Beneath the always embarrassing photograph that freezes one's teenaged awkwardness forever in amber is a quote selected by the graduating student. Sometimes it is something the student has made up herself (*Can't wait to get outta here! Have a great summer!*), and sometimes it is by an eminence like Sophocles (*I conclude that all is well*) or Mark Twain (*Tell me where a man buys his cornpone, and I'll tell you what his 'pinions is*).

A great deal of thought went into my quote since, although not literally written in stone, it would be essentially written in stone, a high school yearbook in its eternal immutability being as close in our era as we have to stone. After an exhaustive search of books, records, movies, and whatever literary and pop detritus I could find, I finally settled on the following lyrics written by the blues singer and guitar player B.B. King:

*Nobody loves me but my mother,*
*And she could be jivin' too,*
*Now you see why I act funny, baby,*
*When you do the things you do.*

Thinking this was a masterstroke, I informed Dad. His response: Your father doesn't love you?

Goodbye, B.B. King.

Looking at the picture of me circa the 70s, there is the onion dome hair, the wide tie, the outdated jacket. And below this adolescent apparition is the quote I wound up using, from Kurt Vonnegut, borrowed from his novel *Slaughterhouse-Five.*

*We on Tralfamadore spend an eternity looking at the pleasant moments. That is what Earthlings should do. Ignore the bad times and concentrate on the good ones.*

I squirm.

Several caveats occur now that I am thirty-seven. Regarded from the perspective of someone who is thirty-seven as opposed to seventeen, it goes without saying that I no longer like it, if I ever did, since it was always a sad substitute for the piece of blues haiku that had crashed and burned on my sensitivity to Dad's sensitivity. If only I hadn't referenced someplace called Tralfamadore, with its scent of pencil-necked geek wearing a *Star Trek* costume while standing in line for some obscure actor's autograph at a comic book convention in San Diego. Moving past Tralfamadore, there is the philosophy elucidated by the quote itself, a call for avoidance. Finally, in its admonition to "ignore the bad times" Vonnegut's words utterly contradict the blues ethic which dictates we embrace the bad times, then get drunk and have sex. As it happens, the perfect quote was there for seventeen-year-old me in the Vonnegut novel, one that in its elegant braiding of fatalism and endurance is perfectly tailored to the inevitable low moments most of us experience, and like so many things when I was young and raw, I missed it.

*So it goes.*

Otis Spann moves me, but when the record ends rather than playing the other side, I remain seated, too enervated to stir. Back in high school the blues were the answer for my troubles, uplifting, transporting. But now that the actual blues (not the pretend-in-your-teenaged-bedroom kind but the kind that accompanies death and heartache) have hit, I would like to say that the music nourishes, it's deep pain gives sonic succor to my tortured soul and delivers me to a place of sweet relief, acceptance, and love. But tonight I can't connect with all the complaining.

I flip to the back of the yearbook where I see the memorial page. A classmate named John died senior year. The lines commemorating him in the book were superimposed on a photograph of gentle waves lapping against a sandy shore, perhaps insensitive given that he had drowned. John made me think of another kid who died the same year. His name was Bruce and he was in the class ahead of me. Bruce was home for the holidays, ingested downers, and, Hendrix-like, choked on his vomit. We had gone to elementary school together so I had known him for what was (for a seventeen-year-old) a long time. The funeral was packed. I stood in the back surrounded by a phalanx of teenagers, each sadder than the next. I remember thinking *I can't believe that's Bruce in the coffin.* We were playing basketball when someone came into the gym and told us he was dead. My first reaction—after shock—was anger. At him. How could he have done that to us? I wonder if people are going to be angry at me. *I'm* angry at me.

I place my yearbook back on the shelf, return to the records, and pull out *My Aim is True* by Elvis Costello. I extract the vinyl and place it on the turntable. The song is "I'm Not Angry."

*I'm not angry, I'm not angry anymore.*

He means it ironically. That is something I connect with. This is what speaks to me now, the anger, the irony. I settle in and listen. The low hum of traffic drifts up from the street. Ordinarily, this is a calming sound but tonight I am seething. I am angry at Dad for having had cancer. I am angry with my mother for having cancer and dying. I am angry that I inherited whatever gene it is that allows this havoc to occur. My anger is hard and resistant, like the pit of a particularly bitter fruit. I think of the doctor who wrote the book that claims cancer patients cause their diseases and I wonder if I'm mad at him because he's so unspeakably wrong or because he's right. Have I given low-grade, follicular mixed cell lymphoma to myself? Is there some inner amalgamation of worry and pain and misplaced pride and unwillingness to face difficult emotions which has combined to form the jokey construct of a personality that resists engagement because vulnerability in my mind equals defeat and I, in my weakness, refuse to be defeated—that causes cancer?

I hope not. Of course not. No.

We are who we are. Our qualities are our qualities. But if our anger, and impatience, and willingness to judge, and oversensitivity, and loathing, and fear are like hairs on a particularly unruly head, perhaps they can be tamed. A tiger will sit on a stool. It's still very much a tiger, but there it is, seated.

\* \* \*

Letting friends know you have what might be a fatal illness is not a subject the etiquette books address. Who gets what information and how much do they get? Who don't you tell? Do you keep the whole thing a secret and explain your new baldness as a style choice? There are many questions to be answered.

I decide to inform a trusted circle. I don't want them to

hear it from each other so I take it upon myself to call them individually. Here is a typical conversation:

> *Hi, it's Seth. I'm fine, you? Yeah, everything's good. Susan's doing great. It's a healthy pregnancy. Allegra's terrific. I just wish she'd sleep through the night. But . . . uhhh . . . there's one little thing. Before I tell you what it is, I want to say that I'm going to be fine. No, no, no. It's not that big a deal. I have cancer.*

(Pause while this information sinks in.)

> *Yeah, lymphoma. I didn't know what it is either, but I do now.*

(Additional pause while they calculate my survival chances.)

> *The lymph system, right. I'm going to have some chemotherapy for a while but my doctor says they can control it. No, I'm doing okay under the circumstances—which aren't that bad! We're really looking forward to the new baby!*

So whom do I tell? Chris and Mary-Paula, John and Laura, Larry, Max, Nina, Barry, Jeff and Meg, Jake, Cliff and Chana, and Leonard, a special case. Why single out Leonard? Because Leonard has his own struggles as the son of a mother that made *Medea* look like an afternoon in daycare, a father who committed suicide, and the brother of a famous comedian. Leonard often calls to tell me jokes, the opposite of what I am doing.

My soft-pedaling still produces gasps through the phone. I try to reassure my friends, to make them laugh. Anytime someone hears you have cancer they're thinking about what they're going to wear to your funeral. They don't want to think this and they're certainly not going to tell you they're thinking it, but people do tend to take a quick peek at the worst-case picture and everyone knows what it is. My friends, to their credit, serve the right combination of platitudes, offer to be of help, do this, get that, be there. But there is nothing for anyone to do or get, no place for them to be. I swear them all to secrecy and hang up the phone with the knowledge that I will go through this mostly with my pregnant wife, and my two-year-old daughter, my brother, and father nearby. And although I invoke Drew and Dad, I know the heaviest burden will fall on Susan.

In the event you are wondering, Leonard handled it well.

It would take someone more evolved than I to sympathize with the people contemplating my "future" which, let's face it, *should* be in quotes. And I know they're having a hard time because even the most hopeful person, when confronted with someone dear to them receiving a cancer diagnosis, hears a little voice in their head that says, *It's curtains.*

Several days later I receive handwritten letters from Chris, an attorney, and Larry, a comedy writer with whom I recently collaborated on a short film. They are two of my closest friends and rarely in our conversations are we addressing matters of life and death, unless it's that of someone we don't know personally. Conversations are the usual soup of sports, or movies, or the aggravations of our professional and personal lives. But never our health and double never our mortality. The letters these guys have written are so authentic and heartfelt as to be completely out of character and I am so touched by the simple gesture that I immediately manage to lose both.

\* \* \*

The Class Notes section of my college alumni magazine provides a reliable source of quarterly amusement when I read about all the weddings, births, and career milestones that fellow alumni want to share. Anticipating my first round of chemotherapy, I draft a letter to the class correspondent:

**Seth Greenland '77**, writes: Life was trundling along pretty well, marriage, career, parenthood, when BAM! Cancer! Stage 4, if you were wondering. I missed our tenth reunion mostly due to lack of interest and now I don't know if I'll be alive for the twentieth. I've lost touch with nearly the entire class. There's a reason for that. I don't even know if any of you remember me at this point which would make sense since most of my friends were in other classes and I don't often think about my college years. So why am I posting this in Class Notes? Good question. We want to be remembered, don't we? To know that we left markers that will remind people who knew us that we were there. Most of us don't get statues; I can pretty much guarantee you that no one in our college class will get a statue unless they commission it themselves. But if you're reading the Class Notes, it's because you want your memory jogged. Who was I to you? Anything? Did we take a class together, live in the same dorm, play pickup basketball, share a bong? Did we have sex? I should probably apologize to anyone with whom I had sex. As an undergraduate I was not a maestro of the female orgasm.

We read some books, wrote papers, took tests; we drank, then drank some more. What I can remember, I remember fondly.

Perhaps more important than the question of who was I to you, is who was I? Our alma mater at the time we attended was culturally dominated by the large percentage of students that had attended prep schools. Our sailing team was always good. Our basketball team—on which I played—less good. While punk bands in motorcycle jackets and torn jeans held together by safety pins raged at CBGB I wore khakis, oxford cloth shirts from Brooks Brothers, and hiking boots. Occasionally, I wore deck shoes. This is mortifying to me now. I was an English major and my favorite author was F. Scott Fitzgerald. So besotted was I with his entire oeuvre, and by oeuvre in this case I mean more than the glittering short stories he wrote and *The Great Gatsby* and the perhaps even superior *Tender Is the Night* but also his expatriate life in Paris, capering in the fountain at the Plaza Hotel, gin-fueled struggles in Hollywood, the combination of cheek and verve with which he became a cultural avatar during a flowering of American dynamism, that during my sophomore year I applied to transfer to Princeton, Fitzgerald's alma mater. They politely declined my offer to attend their university, which is how I came to spend four years with you. I cringe at the callow version of me so perhaps we have that in common.

Senior year I took the law boards. Although I managed to become the editor-in-chief of the college newspaper, it did not occur to me that I could be a writer. I didn't know any writers. As a breed, I held them in awe. The day Kurt Vonnegut materialized on campus to help dedicate the new library and I found myself standing next to him, I was so thrown by his corporeal presence that when I tried to let him know that I had quoted from one of his novels in my high school yearbook the words were rocks in my mouth. After graduating I struggled to forge another identity. And eventually I did. There have been a few good years. I worked in movies and television, wrote some plays. I got married, had a daughter. You and I spent four years together and never really talked.

\* \* \*

The rabbi was dressed in a pink tutu and wearing a pith helmet. And strumming a guitar. Susan and I were living in California and I liked it a lot more the second time. Our kids were attending a great school, our careers thriving, and cancer was increasingly behind me, its primary residue a silt-like gloom that had settled somewhere at the root of my consciousness and stubbornly refused to dissipate.

About the rabbi in the tutu: it was Purim, the holiday where after Jews once again commemorate a tyrant trying to kill us everyone is encouraged to get drunk and make merry. Sometimes this involves costumes; hence, the costume-clad rabbi at our Santa Monica synagogue. What made this instance particularly memorable was that it was witnessed by Susan's brother-in-law and sister who were visiting us in California. This was only the second time they had been in the presence of a rabbi and in the first instance, that rabbi was not wearing a tutu (it was at our wedding and a tutu would have been awkward). They were nonplussed since, as we have established, their small town has no Jews and when the people there imagine Jews the images that come to mind probably don't involve rabbis in tutus and pith helmets.

After much discussion, Susan and I had decided to raise our children Jewish. Reared by a Protestant and a Catholic, she had hoped to forge a compromise by bringing the kids to a Unitarian church. Despite well-known and admirable adherents like Emerson and Thoreau, Unitarianism did not supply the comedy and culinary traditions I required. There were over a billion Christians in the world, the Jews had been decimated, and if we were going to raise ours in any faith, it was the Jews that needed help. To my eternal gratitude, Susan went along with my atavistic declaration. It has not been uncomplicated for her.

For my birth family and me, being Jewish was always more about smoked fish than God. We were what our rabbi called Revolving Door Jews, in at Rosh Hashanah, out at Yom Kippur. Despite the desultory nature of my parents' Judaism, I was forced to attend Sunday school at the Westchester

Jewish Community Center, a gulag of suburban Yiddishkeit. Housed in a sprawling 1950s-style building, the JCC was slightly more spiritual than a trip to Schraft's, a local restaurant known for its spectacular blandness. Uncomfortably attired in coats, ties, and leather shoes that pinched, we small, suburban Semites sat in neat rows where moonlighting public-school teachers hectored us about the glories of the Jewish people. Here is what they taught us: Abraham nearly murders his son, a bush talks to Moses, Noah builds a boat, Joseph gets a coat, and Lot's wife gets turned into a pillar of salt. I wrack my brain to remember anything else I learned there but I am stumped.

Our rabbi was a pompous windbag who comported himself not as if he were God's messenger but, rather, as if *he* were actually God; you would never have seen him in a tutu. The cantor keened as if he was in perpetual, albeit loud, mourning, all five thousand years of Jewish suffering emerging from his throat in one endless, resonant kvetch. Ours was an American world of sitcoms, sports, and the Hardy Boys; everything was the future and the past did not exist, much less the one that involved five millennia of tragedy. These men were from another sphere. The services they led transcended the merely uninspiring; they were funereal. Their version of religion reeked of death, and the stultifying boredom that comes when what you feel is an utter disconnectedness from anything you recognize as having meaning. Judaism, as it turns out, is an organic, evolving belief system that embraces and sanctifies life. It is joyous music and literature and art and comedy and food. The rabbi and the cantor of my youth, bless them, were soul killers with whom I was forced by my parents to check in every Sunday. My once-a-week religious experience felt like a nonsequitur. My parents thought they could drop me off, pick me up three hours later, and check the box marked "Spiritual development."

The Westchester JCC was a large Reform congregation, and to accommodate the overflow during High Holy Day services, we would rent the Westchester County Center, a vast barn of a room, home to boat shows and high school basketball championships. The holy ark would be placed in rough approximation to where one of the hoops would be when basketball was being played. Although my mother was not conventionally religious, she insisted on arriving an hour early to these services so she could get a good seat. This was puzzling, since she did not feel her presence was required at services any other time of year, but we were nonetheless dragged along, voluble protests ignored. Because of our early arrival, my brother and I were so enervated by the time the actual service began, our primary challenge was not atoning for our sins, but staying awake. The rabbi recited the prayers from on high, the cantor unleashed his doleful lamentations, worthies from the community addressed the congregation, organ music played, and I was narcoleptic. Oh, for their services now, their mournful cadences, their soporific intonations. Those two would have me unconscious faster than a general anesthetic.

Along with the High Holy Days, the other event on our annual Jewish calendar was the Passover seder. Every year we would make the traffic-choked pilgrimage to my aunt's split-level house on Long Island. Built in the 1950s and set in a cookie-cutter neighborhood where each house looked the exact same, it was a perfect metaphor for how religion was practiced in my home.

*Why? Because this is how everyone does it, that's why!*

The seder, meant to be a festive meal celebrating the liberation of the Jews from slavery in Egypt, was, in the iteration performed by my extended family, much closer to the enslavement than the liberation. Although I liked my Long Island relatives, Passover was a formal affair in their home and as a rambunctious child this approach did not suit me. Like the captivity of our ancestors, their seder was lengthy and humorless.

After battling the Long Island Expressway, we would eat chopped liver (a highlight), declaim prayers in a language no one in my immediate family spoke a word of, then mercifully get in the car and drive home. During the ride back to Westchester, my father, more irritable than usual from the combination of indecipherable Hebrew and undrinkable Manishewitz, upbraided me for accidentally sticking my knees into his back from my perch on the seat behind him. His back had nerves like naval sonar and could sense knee-to-seat contact before it actually occurred, and it was impossible to relax after these seders until I was in my own bed. So, Passover was like the High Holy Days and Sunday school only with more time in the car. If this is what people meant when they said religion, it was not for me.

It wasn't that I wanted to embrace anything else, although for a time Catholicism beckoned. This is back before I knew the Catholic Church to be a font of anti-Semitism, Holocaust complicity, and institutionalized child molestation. A third-grade classmate named David was Catholic and he attended religious school every Wednesday, something which allowed him to leave Miss Simbonis's class at two o'clock in the afternoon, an hour earlier than we Jews were permitted to go. One day I noticed the textbook the Catholics had given him. Done in comic book style, it was a rendering of the Passion. I quickly flipped through it, admiring the drawings, but began to slow down as the story picked up steam. They placed a crown of *thorns* upon his head. That was impressive, a means of torture I was not familiar with. Jesus had to lug a giant *cross* with a crown of thorns upon his head. Grisly, but appealing to an eight-year-old with a taste for the macabre. They *flagellated* him while he lugged the cross around with the crown of thorns on his head. The word "flagellated" was a mystery but

it certainly sounded like a serious punishment. Then the cruci-
fixion. Talk about a climax! It was riveting, astonishing! They
*nailed* a man to a cross? Who knew what a cross was, but it
looked cool looming over everyone on that hill. Particularly
with Jesus *nailed* to it. Hanging there. With spikes through his
palms and his feet. And two other poor schnooks, one on each
side of him, nailed there, too! So not only was Jesus being tortured to death, but he had company up on that cross of his. It
was a mass killing. And those guys were getting the same treatment from the centurions who had metal hats with what
looked like brooms attached to them. Even the hats in this religious school comic were great. Maybe I could be a centurion
for Halloween!

Some context: I was not a particularly morbid child. But at
the time, I was fascinated by horror movies. *Frankenstein* and
*Dracula* were *ur*-texts, templates for a developing aesthetic.
The carnage and havoc they depicted were deeply seductive. I
built models of the monsters purchased at a hobby shop, painting each individual part carefully, meticulously gluing them
together with the concentration of a watchmaker then giving
them pride of place on my shelf. I was deeply enamored with
this stuff. Thus, the torture of Jesus—that was something I
could relate to. Not in any spiritual way, mind you. The healing of the sick, the walking on water, the Sermon on the
Mount, these things, being congenial, were of scant interest.
But what they unleashed on him was terrific in a Saturday at
the movies kind of way. That he was meant to be dying for the
sins of Man did not enter into my thinking. Although the stories they taught us in Sunday school were hardly without merit,
being exposed to the Jesus narrative made me feel like I had
been drinking chocolate milk my whole life and someone just
poured me a shot of bourbon. To be sure, the Jews were no
slouches when it came to mayhem. Yet didn't God stay
Abraham's knife before he could stab his son? And who were

the people who drowned in the Flood? Who perished when Sodom and Gomorrah were destroyed? The Hebrew Bible contains massacres and I didn't know the victims. But Jesus was the main character of their book and look what happened to him.

Then they topped it.

After the harrowing day Jesus spent hiking through Jerusalem wearing a crown of thorns and dragging that cross around before being crucified, it was surprising that the story kept going. They torture him, he dies, curtain. I desultorily continued through David's Jesus comic, wondering why it wasn't over yet. His mother cries. The disciples are sad. When does this end? Hold on. They eyeball his tomb three days later and lo and behold—he's not there! What happened? Where has he gone? He's been resurrected!

Jesus was a ghost.

That evening, my parents were in bed reading when I came in to say goodnight. I had large questions on my mind, eschatological ones. Why hadn't they told me about this Jesus person? In a neutral tone, my father informed me that Jesus played for the other team. It was like we were Yankee fans and Jesus a Dodger. I considered that for a moment. I knew all about the Dodgers, even liked Sandy Koufax and Maury Wills. But they were not our guys. The Dodgers may have been perfectly acceptable human beings, but we were Yankee fans and that's all there was to it. Then my mother did something I still don't understand. She asked if I wanted to go to Catholic religious school.

My mother grew up in Brooklyn, in a Russian-Jewish family. Her father's name at birth was Isidore Levinovitch, but he "anglicized" it to Irving Levine, which compared to Isidore Levinovitch was Cary Grant. Although my grandfather spent more time with his bookie than his rabbi, he was, in today's parlance, Jewish-identified, as was my grandmother, and my mother's two older sisters. So, for her to raise this question was akin to saying *I would be happy if you married your cousin.*

At the time, I didn't know this but my mother had flirted with Ethical Culture when she was younger and going through a seeker phase. Never mind that the Ethical Culture Society was more or less a front organization for disaffected Jews who believed they could extirpate their inner shtetl by associating themselves with something more anodyne. It represented a refuge for those tired of more traditional approaches to spirituality. Apparently, my mother was once one of those people. It's unlikely she actually would have sent me to Catholic school on Wednesday afternoons with my friend David and I wouldn't have gone anyway. The torture of Jesus may have been my kind of story, but if it involved more school, well, I wasn't *that* interested.

My parents forced me to attend Sunday school until I was confirmed.

*Confirmed.*

As what? A Jew, I suppose, as if that needed confirmation. They even hosted a celebratory gathering at our house for friends and relatives on a Sunday afternoon in the spring. To their eternal credit, they did not force me to have a bar mitzvah so this was their chance to make a public statement about having passed along the legacy. With a stomach full of soda and potato chips, I vowed I was done with religion.

* * *

Reeling from the shock of the diagnosis, I am hopeful the medical community can get the violent putsch in my body under control, thrash the mutating barbarians. But what of the German expressionist painting in my head?

Desperation makes us do strange things.

I reconsider religion.

The traditional approach will not work for me, the one that involves putting on fancy clothes and going into a house of worship. That seems counterintuitive. What I can do is pray. Or more precisely, beg, grovel, and self-excoriate. For someone looking to cultivate these behaviors, working as a writer in Hollywood is an unrivalled training regimen so I know I will be ready. Will I be able to ignore my nonbelief in a sentient God who is remotely aware of my current predicament?

Let's see—

Susan is sleeping when I climb out of bed and bend my knees, putting first one foot, then the other behind me. The floor is hard; the position unnatural. I am kneeling. Never mind that Jews don't kneel. Kneeling is Catholic. But it adds to the idea of supplication to be supplicating from your knees so here I am, secular New Yorker on a rigid unforgiving floor, having abandoned self-respect, getting ready to beg.

*Dear God.* Oh, that's original. *You are the intelligence in the cosmos, the order and the pattern.* Too much? *You are the lost chord that must be rediscovered if harmony is to be achieved.* All right, that's not bad. *It is You who animates our spirit and weaves our soul into the fabric of the universe. Who am I to You? I know if You were talking to me at a party, You would already be looking over my shoulder. If You got another call while we were having a telephone conversation, You would take it. This does not bother me though, since I am hardly sure that You even exist.* Maybe I shouldn't mention that while I'm praying. *I used to think You were an old man with a big white beard who wore a Tyrolean hat.* How can I possibly expect Him to take me seriously after I say I envisioned Him in a Tyrolean hat? *In my mind you were Swedish or Belgian, some kind of northern European, but not Slavic because they hate the Jews and definitely not a Jew Yourself or why would You treat the Jews like shit? The Inquisition AND the Holocaust?*

*Seriously?* Perhaps I should not have mentioned the Jews since I think He actually might be anti-Semitic. *I know You are unknowable which I understand is a paradox but I must try and comprehend it. You are what we strive toward. I wonder if You ever get tired of listening to terrified agnostics trying to pray.* Did I have to mention that I'm an agnostic? Is that supposed to help? *We beg and flatter and cajole and every ounce of it comes from fear. But You must already know that. You're great, I'll always be good, and if I fail I'll try to do better, please, I'm begging You, don't kill me. And if you do, then you can go fuck yourself.*

*Amen.*

Back in bed I marvel that I am able to do something so completely out of character. *That* has to be good.

Susan stirs and asks me if I'm all right. Promise me, I say, that if I live through this we'll visit Varanasi. That's where they burn the bodies on the banks of the Ganges River, isn't it? Yes, it is. She wants to know why I'd like to go there of all places. Varanasi is a deeply spiritual city, one that is sacred in the Hindu tradition, a place to which someone who claims to be agnostic should not be drawn. Because if we're watching the bodies be cremated, I tell her, it means we're alive. Fine, she says, we'll go to Varanasi if that's what you want. And then she rolls over and goes back to sleep and the unquiet dreams that are dreamed by a young, pregnant lawyer whose husband might be dying. I stare at the ceiling and think about burial versus cremation and the music the mourners played at Lester Young's funeral. The family of Young's estranged wife refused to let his close friend Billie Holiday perform. Billie Holiday would be welcome at my funeral. The life lessons imparted in the smoke of her voice remain timeless.

Perhaps prayer would come more easily in a religion that worshipped Billie Holiday.

*  *  *

What am I doing parked on a plastic chair in a bare-walled room masturbating in the middle of the afternoon? And who has not asked themselves that exact question?

This story begins in a juice bar around the corner from our apartment. Before today I had never entered this establishment. A bar is where you order whiskey. A juice bar? Not for me.

Until now.

Because—cancer. It has catapulted me out of my comfort zone.

I am staring at a shot of wheatgrass juice—it looks remarkably unappetizing—that has just been placed in front of me when Susan asks, "How do you feel about masturbating into a cup?"

"What?"

"I want us to go to a fertility clinic."

"But why? We already have a daughter. And you're four months pregnant. That's plenty of kids right there."

"Just in case," Susan replies. Then, one of her favorite phrases, "Belt and suspenders."

A long pause. I look away.

She ups the ante: "We'll buy porn."

I'm not particularly interested in porn. Porn is not the point.

I toss back the shot of wheatgrass juice. It tastes vile, like licking a frog. Going to a fertility clinic is unappetizing in the extreme, porn-laden or porn-less. It is just an additional humiliation, one more station of the cross of cell mutation which, despite its pleasing iambic pentameter, is depressing.

I have always been a little disturbed by the idea of nontraditional conception. I am not proud of this because I know many people who have gone through the infertility rigmarole and the pain that accompanies the experience. I salute them and their children. But test tubes and turkey basters have always been a bit science fiction for me, not something I would voluntarily engage in.

However.

That was then. This is important to Susan and she seems thrilled with the idea. It's proactive, forward-looking. Since I am riddled with guilt (not to mention cancer) at the possibility that I might die on her, I agreed to go.

Masturbation is an act most people have engaged in, but few want to sing about. There are many bugaboos attached to the act of pleasuring oneself in our society and they find amusing form in the punishment predicted for those who engage in this pastime. Blindness and hair on the palms, Biblical in their extremity, are two of the more common afflictions thought to await those who bring themselves to climax solo and parents, hawk-eyed, are on alert for a toddler's furtive hand dip into his or her pants. Who knows how common masturbation really is but I suspect that it ranks somewhere between blinking and breathing.

I can unequivocally state that I am pro-masturbation. This probably disqualifies me for public office in our great nation. In that sense, it's like being an atheist. Godlessness and masturbation walk hand in hand in America, two outlaws condemned to wander the fruited plain, vilified and alone. Let me cast my political future to the winds and say when it comes to masturbation, I am a believer. Not an exponent, nor one that attempts to convert people. I just think individuals should be allowed to masturbate and not have a big deal made out of it as long as they're not sitting next to me on the crosstown bus.

Here's another doctor joke told to me by my friend Leonard:

A guy walks into a doctor's office. The doctor looks at him and says, You have to stop masturbating. The guy asks why and the doctor says, So I can examine you.

What does masturbation have to do with cancer? This is the result of Susan having asked Dr. Speyer what happens to the male reproductive ability after chemotherapy, specifically, what happens to the patient's sperm. You will recall it causes problems.

And now we find ourselves on yet another gorgeous day in late spring standing in front of an inconspicuous brownstone on 30th Street between First and Second avenues. The place is called Repro and it is situated on the ground floor. Susan looks at me. Her glance says, Why aren't you moving? Again, as if this is a rerun of my performance in front of Memorial Sloane Kettering, I am riveted to the sidewalk, only this time my fingers are wrapped around a magazine that contains photographs of naked women. Now her eyes are saying, Will you go in or do I have to drag you?

When it comes to pornography, we have established that I am at best indifferent, so none was handy at home. I have no idea what is provided in terms of stimulation at Repro but sense it will be like a doctors' office and I didn't think I could get my groove on with nothing to stimulate me but an old copy of *Reader's Digest*. For this reason, we stopped at a newsstand. There was a cornucopia of pornography available, publications for every taste and fetish. I purchased the copy of *Playboy* currently in my hand. Why? Because I always associate *Playboy* with being twelve years old. This is the age when contraband copies circulated like *samizdat* among horny preadolescents who had never laid eyes on the body of an actual woman. The pictorials, party jokes, cartoons, and especially the centerfolds were a collective holy sexual grail, signifiers of what awaited us in an adulthood filled with nothing but sports cars, women's breasts, and not having to worry about concepts like objectification. If a kid managed to sneak his dad's issue out of the house and make it to the playground undetected, he was a conquering hero. *Playboy* carries me back to this time in my life, so much more innocent, optimistic; so much more exalted than the period I am enduring now.

The *Playboy* I purchased has a series of photographs of a model currently appearing in a national advertising campaign. I will hold it in abeyance, keep my powder dry.

Somehow, this feels even weirder than going into Memorial Sloan Kettering where all I had to do was listen to a doctor tell me that I was probably going to die. What awaits me at Repro is more mortifying. Susan tugs my arm. Clutching my porn like a teddy bear, I follow her into the building. The waiting area is bright and bland. To my relief, no one bursts into laughter when I walk through the door. Susan is acting like we are going to the post office. As if there is nothing unusual about what we are here to do. It is impossible for me to know what is going on in her head at this moment. It does not occur to me to ask because I am a balloon, ready to float away in a cloud of angst and vanish into the sky. She is the string that secures me to the ground. Were it not for her, I would be rising through the Earth's atmosphere right now.

A matter-of-fact male nurse gives me a form to fill out. He barely makes eye contact. That I am about to go off and masturbate into a cup because I have cancer and my wife thinks I might wind up sterile if not dead does not concern this man. I give him the form, and he points down a hallway. I smile ruefully at Susan and proceed with my *Playboy* into a small room equipped with dog-eared copies of down-market porno magazines like *Nugget* and *Chic*—who curated these selections?—a small video monitor, and several beat-up cassettes with no labels. What are they? *Masturbation for Beginners? The Little Mermaid?* I check that the door is locked. Everyone that observed my entrance knows what I'm here to do and no one would be surprised should they walk in on me, but still, who wants to suffer that particular humiliation? A video goes in and, feeling utterly ludicrous, I drop my pants and press play.

The exercise feels futile. It is bad enough I am here at all, that I am being subjected to third-rate porn is truly depressing, a further turning of the knife that could send a more sensitive person in a Sylvia Plath direction.

I think about how these performers wound up in the porn video here at Repro. Clearly, this was not what they had in mind when starting out. Surely, they dreamed of other things, but here they are, in this sad and tawdry production. So often life does not turn out the way people expect. If I have to endure the indignity of this process, where is my seraglio, my gang of nubile concubines to extract the precious, pre-chemo seed in the most timeless manner?

In my overactive imagination, that's where.

Here I am, sick and scared, in a cheerless room watching sex between couples who look like they were recruited at the Port Authority bus station on Eighth Avenue in the late 70s. Watching them is like viewing a nature documentary about skanky baboons. I turn to the magazines and choose one from the table. It is funky to the touch, with a greasy sheen, and I am already feeling put-upon. I'm not going to revel in degradation. Enough with the Repro-supplied stimuli. Out comes *Playboy*. There is that model from the national ad campaign. I am happy to see her. She is smiling and buxom, but not over-weight, arrayed like a fertility goddess on a hay bale, head thrown back, laughing, carefree. Are those implants? They must be. No matter. I will love them.

I manage to achieve tumescence and then we are having sex, the two of us, the model from the national ad campaign and I on the hay bale, hot and torrid, transporting, beyond the four-walled institutional room, and Repro, and the East Thirties, above Manhattan and up through the soft clouds and into the blue beyond where we float weightless and free over the shimmering world for a few blissful moments and I forget everything that binds me to the earth and its vale of tears, so when the Fourth of July arrives in my cerebellum I salute America and fill the sample cup.

The power of the mind is astonishing.

As I pull my pants up and fasten my belt, I feel like a sex worker. It is my least favorite act of autoeroticism ever.

*Ever.*

I arrived in the room to do a job, the job is done, and now it is time to leave. But first I affix my name to a label and place it on the cup. I enter the waiting area and have the horrifying thought that everyone there is thinking, hey, *that* guy just finished jacking off. Of course, that would have been like a waitress at a diner thinking, hey, *that* guy just ate waffles. But the reader understands where I am with shame at this point in the story and knows I am self-conscious about walking around with the sperm cup like it's a spritzer at a cocktail party. I hand it to the male nurse and try to pretend that this is normal. He takes it and writes something down on a clipboard. I have just masturbated not thirty feet from him yet he and I have an unspoken agreement to act as if I have spent the previous ten minutes playing Donkey Kong. He tells me to return the next day to repeat the process.

I have to come back?

Susan gets up from her chair and smiles at me. It's once again difficult to imagine what she has been thinking while patiently sitting in the waiting area as her cancer-riddled husband "pleasures" himself in the next room. I don't want to ask.

"Thank you," she says. She puts her arm around my waist as we walk out of the clinic. Her touch is enveloping and secure. For a moment, I feel safe.

It is said the Inuit people have twenty-eight words for snow, since it is such an important component of their lives. Our culture has at least fifty synonyms for masturbation.

Make of that what you will.

\* \* \*

I have steeled myself for the ordeal ahead of me, informed my friends, masturbated into a cup. As my cells continue to enthusiastically replicate I want nothing so much as a drink. The news is sinking in. The muckety-mucks do not disagree. There has been no misdiagnosis, no mistake in the lab. No tap on the shoulder where someone says *Joking!* No *deus ex machina.* Where is a double scotch? There's a bottle of Johnnie Walker Black in the pantry.

Do I have the drink?

Susan ordinarily likes a glass of wine, but since she is pregnant Chardonnay is a no-go zone. Under the circumstances, I can't believe she's not guzzling pitchers of margaritas, but right now? A model of self-control. Frankly, who could blame her if she got completely plastered?

"Would you like some wine with dinner?" she asks me.

"I would love a glass of wine, but no thanks."

"Why not? You could use a glass."

What can be controlled? Food has always been something I've loved and no matter how much I ate, I never gained weight. And I was indiscriminate in my consumption: steak, ribs, pork chops, pizza, lasagna, spaghetti, roast beef, bacon, ham, turkey, chicken, salads, potatoes, white rice, noodles, Chinese food, Indian food, Thai food, Japanese food, Mexican food. In other words, pretty much anything.

Now, in an attempt to assert some kind of mastery, I perform a review of my intake. From a cursory reading of newspapers and magazines, I am dimly aware of the chemical content of much of the animal protein we consume. It is becoming widely known that hormones, chemicals, and additives with unpronounceable names are being zealously pumped into the chicken and beef we ingest routinely. Following the initial foray into the literature of cancer, I dip a tentative toe into the literature of healthy eating. The consensus among the healthy eaters is simple: meat and chicken are bad. In my overwrought state, I consider the level of hormones and chemicals and additives in beef and poultry and think it's a wonder everyone who eats them doesn't drop dead on the spot or grow chicken wings on their neck.

"I'm not eating chicken or beef anymore," I announce to Susan.

She looks at me neutrally. "Okay."

"I'm not ready to swear off fish."

"We can eat fish if you want."

"And I don't think I can be macrobiotic at this point."

"I'm getting a macrobiotic cookbook. It'll be fun."

Fun? Oh, god. Now I really need that drink. But I have decided to forswear drinking. I enjoy drinking and have long admired the great alcoholic writers. Alcoholism is a far better tragic flaw than hubris, the one favored by the ancient Greeks. Hubris, for the classics-deprived, is excessive pride, as in *pride cometh before a fall*. Drinks, too, often cometh before a fall— down a staircase for instance. But no one ever bothered to coin that phrase.

What do I think I am going to prove by not drinking?

\* \* \*

These days, I don't drink much. A few glasses of the wrong red wine can leave me with a hangover that lasts longer than the American invasion of Grenada. But for eighteen months back in the early 90s I quit. This period included a trip to France (in the worthy footsteps of Dr. Moscowitz) where I was sorely tested. For the purposes of this book, I'd like to write that I was an alcoholic consuming a fifth of Scotch or a case of beer a day, that I was brushing my teeth with vodka and sipping an entire bottle of brandy after dinner, that I was draining bathtubs full of Chianti in Tuscany, or swimming in a vat of Sancerre in France. But that was someone else, someone who was having a far better time than I.

My parents were drinkers. This may come as something of a surprise since Jews are generally not known for their drinking prowess, but that is simply a misrepresentation. I am terrible with money, but a Jew. How can this be so? I have no idea, although my accountant, who is of Irish extraction, wishes it were not the case because my inadequacy as a manager of my own finances makes his job more difficult during tax season. I *wish* I controlled the world. But that rumor of Jewish control is only that, as far as I know—a sour rumor. If there is truly a group of Jews who control the world, I am not on their email list. But if for some reason I am mistaken, and the *Protocols of the Elders of Zion* are correct, please take note, cabal members: contact me so I can join your ranks.

My father was in the advertising business back when smoking and drinking were considered indoor sports and his most important accounts were liquor brands. As such, he felt drinking was his duty. As someone who stood by her husband in all his endeavors, my mother believed she should share this burden. Every night before dinner, Dad poured himself a generous glass of Scotch on the rocks and my mother would have one of her "very, very dry" martinis, a polite way of saying please just wave the bottle of vermouth over the gin. Because straight gin was something a blowsy broad would order in a dockside bar before decamping with the fleet. A martini, on the other hand, with its evocation of a gilded postwar era of sophisticated nightclubs, men in sharp suits smoking cigars, and high-heeled women wearing Chanel while Tony Bennett crooned in the background, was what someone like my mother would drink, even if it was "very, very dry." My father did business in the age of what is fondly remembered as the "three-martini lunch." This is hard to conceive of today, when if someone orders even a single martini at lunch she is being shipped off to rehab by dessert (which no one orders either— it's just a figure of speech). But years ago brave men and women would go forth to lunch and routinely drink themselves stupid before returning to the office where they would perform the duties of an afternoon in varying degrees of inebriation. And this was considered normal. And if, like Dad, you were in the liquor business, it was not only normal, but expected and encouraged.

Having defeated the Nazis and polio, then enacted civil rights legislation and invented color television, no one would argue that this generation was not entitled to a few whiskies before the sun dropped below the yardarm. What have we baby boomers done in comparison? Starbucks? Online poker? Around the time Dad turned fifty he became a serious oenophile and began collecting fine wines. He bought a storage locker/refrigerator which he installed in the basement not far from the bumper pool table and began to keep a wine diary. He would meticulously record each bottle he consumed and describe it as artfully as he could manage using a selection of adjectives with which I was not familiar at the time. Flinty, Fruity, Full, Leafy, Meaty, Mellow, and Moldy (all names a bibulous Walt Disney might have used for the Seven Drunk Dwarfs) were not words that could describe anything that had ever crossed my lips, but they were routinely tossed around our dinner table. When I was fifteen, I was enlisted as a wine taster and allowed to add my expanding descriptive powers to the journal. It was in this context I learned the word "bouquet" in its nonfloral context, and where I first heard the expression "good head," slightly incongruous in retrospect. Dad taught me how to taste wine, really *taste* it, roll it around on the tongue and chew it before swallowing. All of this ceremony seemed comical to me, not to say slightly pretentious, but I played along since I enjoyed drinking wine and being treated like a grown-up.

Our family dinners, the whiskey and gin chased by the fine wine, and the alcohol only partially absorbed by my mother's cooking, could be raucous. My parents became more animated as the liquor flowed, and my mother, in particular, would become livelier, her stories more expansive. She would go on and on, embellishing, occasionally losing her place, always with great good humor. Her narrative plane would be circling the airport for so long sometimes that I would have to remind her to bring it in for a landing. But when I remarked to my father years later that I had observed, occasionally, that he and my mother would get lit at dinner, he was insulted. He had only been drunk once in his life, he assured me. It was in 1941 when Jerry Koegel, with whom he had grown up in the Bronx, was killed while flying a training mission in Washington State. He got blotto, stinking, wild drunk. *That* is what it means to be drunk, he explained. Your mother and I never got drunk.

If that was the definition, maybe *he* never got drunk like that again.

But I did.

I started drinking when I was a sophomore in high school. I wanted to be a drinker, liked the idea of being a drinker. My problem was this: I didn't like to actually drink. I liked the romance, the history, the seeming adultness of it, just not the taste, which was revolting. So, the hard stuff was out. Wine was what you drank with your parents. That left beer. One Friday night sophomore year, my friends Chris, Dave, and I procured three six-packs of Rheingold and repaired to the local duck pond to drink them. My first buzz arrived with beer #3 and I pushed through the entire six-pack because, and I'm not proud to admit this, that's what Chris and Dave were doing. It would have been unmanly to not consume the entire six-pack. For such reasons wars are fought, although at the time I did not have that particular insight. I staggered home, fell asleep, and woke up with my first hangover, a skull rattler that felt as if someone was repeatedly bringing a sledgehammer down on my head.

A driver's license opened up the world of bars. There was a joint adjacent to the railroad station in the next town over, called Danny's. Ordinarily a place for doleful commuters who didn't want to go home after sloshing out of the bar car on the evening train, it attracted an underage clientele because of their willingness to serve virtually anyone. You didn't even need a fake ID. No one cared. It was at Danny's that I discovered the tequila sunrise, the emblematic mixed drink of that era, what the Tom Collins or the sloe gin fizz had been to our parents' generation. With its vivid red, orange, and yellow palette, and candied taste, it was the perfect cocktail for a sixteen-year-old, a knockout punch wrapped in a rainbow. I drank a lot of them. Then I would stuff my face with beer nuts and for the first time in my life experience warm, fuzzy feelings toward people I didn't especially like.

I went to Danny's a lot.

When I was a freshman in college a bar opened on the campus. Dark, noisy, filled with women and their pheromones. I was there every night. While Steely Dan or Al Green blasted on the sound system we drained pitcher upon pitcher of cold draft beer and contrived new ways to recruit sex partners. Occasionally, those plans would be successful. But you could *always* count on getting soused. During my freshman year, if I wasn't drunk every night it was only because I had the flu in March.

I spent that summer on Cape Cod sharing an apartment above a garage with three classmates from college. Despite the Biblical proscription against shellfish, I was working as a lobster fisherman. I had prevailed upon a laconic old salt named Connie Holmes to hire me on his boat, a forty-five-footer which sailed out of Harwich Port, near the elbow on the south side of the Cape. Connie was a man of remarkably few words.

Probably in his late fifties at the time, he had been lobstering his whole life. The other hand on the boat was named Russ. A little older than I, his communication skills mirrored Connie's. No one would mistake this boat for the Algonquin Round Table.

We loaded up with traps and bait then headed out to sea. The work was back-breaking and boring. On the voyage to the fishing area, every available surface was covered in stacks of lobster pots. Piles of boxes stuffed with the frozen fish used as bait were in the cabin with us and when they began to thaw the stench of the decomposing fish was nauseating. We would bait the traps and shove them over the side, one following the other in rapid movement, all hitched together by rope like a giant aquatic charm bracelet. The rope swept the deck at vicious speed and if it caught your ankle, you could be flipped overboard like a potato chip. I got snared my first time out but escaped with a rope burn. Connie and Russ looked at me like I was an imbecile.

When the wood traps became waterlogged, they were dead weight, and pulling them up in the rough seas required superhuman effort. We threw them on the deck and removed the catch. Then we inserted little wedges at the upper hinge of the lobsters' claws and tossed them in a locker. The unfortunate crabs who had wandered into the traps were impaled on the wood spikes at the center of each trap before we pitched it back into the sea. Apparently, crabs are discerning enough to see their dead brethren and think better of going after the bait meant to lure the lobsters. I didn't enjoy killing the crabs summarily, but this is what you do on a lobster boat. It wasn't as if I could discuss my qualms with Connie and Russ. And the money was bad. It wasn't meant to be, but Connie cheated me.

Against this background I called a girl I had met on a ski trip, two years earlier when we were both in high school. Alison lived in Hyannis Port and I thought, since I was in the neighborhood, and it was the 1970s, we would rekindle our holiday-forged friendship. She seemed happy enough to hear from me and we made a date. When the evening arrived, I had the foresight to purchase a pint of cheap tequila, a beverage I was now happy to drink without the sunrise mixer that traditionally accompanied it. I picked Alison up at her family home, a large sprawling house, and we went to a local club where a band was playing. It pains me to say I snuck the tequila into the club but since the cagey Connie Holmes had only paid me a fraction of what was owed, I was on a tight budget. Alison was beautiful, if a little bland, and not much of a conversationalist. She would have fit right in on the lobster boat. Since my desire to be physically intimate with someone declines in direct proportion to their ability to be engaging, after about half an hour it was looking like a long evening. But tequila to the rescue! I managed to purloin a pint glass and, placing it beneath the table, surreptitiously emptied the bottle into it.

Life immediately began to improve. As the night wore on, I sipped the tequila and the music got better, Alison became fascinating, a veritable New England Tina Fey, her every banal utterance a scintillating bon mot, and the entire evening took on a pulsing glow. A pint of tequila will make a person quite drunk and when I escorted Alison out the door of the club and to the car I was far beyond the legal limit. I drove her home without incident and said a quick goodnight, wanting to do nothing more than get back to my apartment and slip into a coma. I was drunk enough that not having sex this evening was going to be a positive outcome.

I turned my car away from Alison's house and down her quiet street, trying to remember how to get home. Left or right, I couldn't recall. But there was Main Street. That had to be good. I turned on to Main Street, happy to have found my way, stepped on the gas, and headed toward Route 6, the main artery of Cape Cod. This would be an amusing story, my reunion with Alison, the bottle of tequila—wait, what were those flashing blue-red lights in my rear window?

The cop, a young dough-faced guy with a police-issue mustache, pulled me over and asked if I knew I was going the wrong way on a one-way street. And since it was Main Street, this was a significant problem. He asked to see my license and registration. Drunker than a fraternity party, but determined to behave like a paragon of rectitude, I quickly produced my license then fumbled for the registration in the glove compartment. He gave them a cursory glance before requesting that I get out of the car. I obeyed, trying to not sway like a palm tree in the night breeze. The cop asked me to touch the end of my nose with the tip of my index finger, a move I executed with considerable aplomb. Then he asked me to walk in a straight line, placing one foot directly in front of another. A lot of people are not able to perform this maneuver stone sober but there I was doing it, I thought, balletically—although not balletically enough to prevent me from being arrested immediately. The cop ordered me to put my hands behind my back and, lo and behold, I was cuffed. Tightly. Uncomfortably. Not having sex with Alison had turned into a far bigger problem than I had anticipated.

Ensconced in the rear of the patrol car, I suavely asked "Do you have any idea who I am?" To this day, I am not sure what made me say this. I know. Obviously, it was the alcohol. But I'm not sure why it made me say this particular thing since I was less than no one, a college kid working a local job for the summer, not rich or famous, or a member of a prominent family. I was just a nineteen-year-old jerk operating a motor vehicle while under the influence of a pint of tequila which had done me no good with Alison. Still, I persisted in this line of questioning. "Do you have any *idea*?" I inquired. The cop in the front seat was intelligent enough to not answer. I can imagine what he was thinking: Yes, I know who you are. You are an entitled jackass who is so drunk it looks like you might throw up all over your white polo shirt but I will not dignify your belligerent question with a response.

The police officer, a profoundly patient man, brought me to the station house. Upon my middle-of-the-night arrival, I looked around and asked the four cops I saw, What are you guys doing here? Why aren't you out catching criminals? The witticisms just flying out of my mouth. The cops barely looked up. This indifference did not deter me. Like a demented entertainer, happily oblivious of the degree to which his act is bombing, I tried again: There must be something better you officers can do than just sitting around.

Still, nothing.

I was booked and informed I would be spending the night. Just like in the movies, they told me I could make one phone call. I called my roommates, thinking they would come down and get me out. Why I thought this, I have no idea but it probably has something to do with being extremely drunk. No one had said anything to me about bail or being released. Still, someone should know I'd been arrested and it was not going to be my parents. The roommate who picked up the phone reacted nonchalantly to the news. It was as if the call had been to say I'll be late to dinner. Even in my current state, that was a surprise. He wished me good luck and then the conversation was over and I was staring at the receiver in my hand. My belt and wallet were confiscated. Then I was deposited in a cell, the door clanging shut behind me. I looked around. There was a metal bed attached to the wall with no bedding, and a metal toilet. Other than that, the cell was empty.

Taking stock of the disaster that had befallen me, I began to scream. Not in fear or alarm. I was way too intoxicated to be scared. I wanted their attention. I did some more variations on the theme of *Do you know who I am?* then moved along to *You are really going to regret this* before concluding with *If you let me go now I'm willing to forget the whole thing.*

Despite my Lincoln-like rhetorical skills, the cell door remained locked. They didn't even offer me a sandwich. After my pathetic attempts to negotiate my freedom had been exhausted, I crumpled on the metal bed and tried to pass out. Because of the amount of tequila consumed prior to my misadventure, this did not prove to be a problem. I drifted off uneasily. My sleep was hard and dreamless.

To say I was startled to wake up a jail cell would be to considerably understate my reaction. A thunderous hangover did not help and meant that my surprise and dismay were marbled with severe physical pain. The morning light stabbed through the slit of the one eye I managed to open like the point of a dagger. Head throbbing, starving and humiliated, I remembered every detail of the previous evening and even at the tender age of nineteen knew enough to be utterly galled by how I had comported myself. I felt profound gratitude the police hadn't come into my cell and pummeled me to oblivion. And along with this gratitude, there was a dusting of shame since no one in my family was the type to wake up in a jail cell.

My mother would not have considered this to be at all appropriate.

After what seemed like an interminable length of time that was probably about an hour, I was taken out of the cell and brought to the local courthouse to be arraigned. There was a holding cell where I was placed with the other miscreants, a pretty tame bunch on Cape Cod (most of them were wearing at least one item from the L.L. Bean catalogue), and we bided our time until called to see the judge, a middle-aged white man with dark hair and black-framed glasses. The defendant who preceded me was also charged with driving under the influence. He was a chucklehead in his twenties and appeared to be local. When the judge asked him why he had been driving, he replied, Because I was too drunk to walk. His impertinence was admirable, but the judge was not amused. The comedian was given a court date and it was my turn. When I took my place in front of the magistrate I noticed there was a group of kids from nearby summer camp there that day. They were on a field trip to the courthouse to see how the criminal justice system works. There was the kindly judge, and there was the jury box, and who's that? The Defendant. Me. I wanted to say to them *No, there's been a mistake, I'm not a defendant.* But I couldn't because there hadn't been and I was.

The judge assigned me a court date and I was released on my own recognizance. I hitchhiked to where the police had taken my car and got it back. Then I drove to Harwich Port where I found my roommates spackled on the furniture. When I asked about their low-key reaction to my phone call, one of them informed me that they had been tripping and my predicament had bummed them out.

At least that explained their nonchalant reaction.

Still considering acceding to my father's wishes and going to law school, I thought it best that it not be known I'd been pinched for a DUI. This is when I learned the phrase "sealed and expunged." I learned this from the Hyannis Port lawyer I paid every dollar I earned that summer to help me navigate my way through the Massachusetts legal system. Thus, there is no record of an arrest, or a night in jail. What little street cred it gives me is utterly unverifiable. But I will swear that it's true. Even after a couple of drinks.

\* \* \*

In conversation, when the word *bone* occurs, I want it to be preceded by words like *chicken* or *lamb* so when Dr. Speyer announces that before treatment begins, a bone marrow extraction is required, it is an unappetizing development. I don't want to contemplate bones because of the skeletal implications. To consider the superstructure that undergirds all of us is to find oneself ruminating on the ephemeral nature of existence. Bones are like a team of oarsmen rowing down the Harlem River in an eight-person shell. If you notice the third one from the bow seat, it's not because that rower is doing something right. In this new context, I worry that anything involving the word *bone* is going to be painful in the extreme. Nonetheless, I recline on a table in Dr. Speyer's examination room. My palms are clammy. But a needle is only a needle. I hitch my shirt up a little and drop my pants slightly, leaving exposed flesh at my lower back, nerve endings minding their own business. The doctor anesthetizes the area with a little jab that I barely feel. This is going to be a breeze, I tell myself. No one has ever described a bone marrow aspiration to me but how bad can it be?

I don't want to see what he's going to put back there—the needle that will penetrate my skin and then my bone—but I find myself peeking over my shoulder. It is a syringe that looks like it is meant for an elephant, comically large, a circus prop, something that should be administered by a cartoon character.

Facing forward again, I settle into the table to await my fate. Nervousness creates a tingling sensation in my WHAT THE?!—a horse has kicked me violently on the right side of my lower back and I am instantly teleported to an uncharted world of pain. Speyer has become Mengele and he is pressing on me with all of his weight, shoving a metal rod into the area two inches to the right of my spine, bloody murder screams of nerve endings ringing in my ears. The pain is so intense, so complete and nullifying it blocks out everything else, the room, the fiend behind me, the light; it explodes in my brain, fires synapses like cannons as the cold metal rips through tissue, penetrates my bone, takes a ravenous bite, chews, swallows, burps, and withdraws.

Adrift in a miasma of sheer, horrific sensory overload. "Motherfucker," I eloquently spit, unable to think of anything else. I want to cry. Then the pain mercifully vanishes as quickly as it arrived. This is disorienting. A second ago an agony unlike anything I had ever experienced. My cheek, moist with perspiration, sticks to the paper on the examination table.

A few silent moments during which I collect myself.

Sitting up, I ask Dr. Speyer if it is weird for him to treat me after he had treated my mother. He assures me that it is not. My parents invited him to a few social occasions and he had accepted. It was their way of trying to appease the gods. Now he informs me he was angry at my father who cut him off when my mother died. I tell him I never thought he had done anything other than all he could. This is not the time to insert myself into whatever psychodrama has developed between him and Dad.

Then the doctor performs another bone aspiration, this one two inches to the left of my spine. The pain is magnificent, transcendent; I am a medieval martyr, my suffering glorious, transported to a realm where everything has been cleansed by the grief of my senses.

When the ordeal is over I return to the fertility clinic where, once again, I masturbate into a cup.

Practice makes perfect.

At home there is a letter from Susan's parents. We have not been close and I appreciate the gesture. My eyes widen as I read the letter. Here is what they say:

We hope you make the most of the time you have left.

*The time you have left.*

This is not what I need right now, these coded "good wishes" with their *you're dying* implication. I write back and thank them for their concern. I sign the letter *Love, Seth*. It's passive-aggressive.

\* \* \*

Waiting for chemo to begin is what I imagine the pre-dawn mustering of troops must have been like before the Battle of Gettysburg. The possibility of death is inescapable, like smoke in a confined space, and all you can do is try not to imagine it. At this point, what is there to talk about?

Memorial Day weekend at Dad's country house in the manicured woods north of the city, the kind of exurban forest etched with dirt roads traveled by late model Mercedes sedans leased to insider traders. Treatment starts Monday and this is a peaceful environment in which to pass the uneasy time. On a happier afternoon not quite three years earlier, Susan and I got married in the backyard. Friends and family, toasts, dancing to a live band assembled by a musician friend for the occasion. The wedding seems like a long time ago. The house is a boxy modern number on a hill overlooking a discreet lake daubed with waterlilies and when my parents bought it ten years earlier my mother supervised a complete renovation. Her presence is everywhere, even if she is not. This casts a further pall on the gloomy holiday weekend. Her essence, though, is in the furniture she selected; the supple and stylish Italian leather sofas in the living room, the circular silver coffee table that we call "the orb." It is in the art on the walls, the modern sculptures, the rustic pottery. It is in the kitchen she designed and the Spanish country dishes with which she stocked it, brightly hued in yellows, blues, and reds. Everything simple, refined but unpretentious. Her spirit palpable.

The less refined element—my father, brother, and I—are settled in the den where we usually chinwag, drink beer, and eat thin-crust pizza with extra garlic from DiNardo's. Susan and Allegra are elsewhere in the house. The TV is off, the large screen an empty void; no one is hungry. Here we are, staring into the middle distance, furtively glancing at each other, uncharacteristically silent. I'm wearing jeans and a tee shirt. The two of them, golf shirts and pressed pants. Actually, Drew's pants are not pressed, something that would have vexed our mother, a believer in rules. Shoes shined, pants pressed. Drew and Dad are golf enthusiasts, the kind who believe golf is actually a sport. I could never be convinced a sport is something you can do while sipping a gin and tonic, an observation they have never found amusing. Tall and lithe, with an athletic physique, Drew is an excellent golfer, our father less so, but both are equally enthusiastic about the game. It is a perfect day for them to be out on the links but, flummoxed by my diagnosis, they choose to be at my side as I contemplate the abyss. We silently prognosticate, ponder the thinkable and unthinkable. I hope that my situation will not devolve. That there will be no bedside moments, me propped on pillows performing bravery in the role of the noble one expiring before his time, pale, paler, palest, the slow fade. Brave would be a stretch. Noble? Please.

The presence of my father and brother keeps me from barking with anxiety. Between intermittent nervous chatter, quiet booms through the airy rooms. Drew and I did not grow up in this house but as adults we spent many Sunday afternoons here with our parents. We talked about which quarterback was better than another, or work, or what a fool some politician was. Our vocabulary, our familiar world, one of conflict and resolution and there's always tomorrow. Conversations between us spark and thrust. They also rarely plunge toward the depths. Not that I want to plumb any great psychological depths at this darkling hour, even if we could. Today the usual river of surface verbiage is dammed. No one knows what to say. The idea of Tomorrow has become unfixed.

From a generation where the masculine ideal required an absence of emotion, Dad is reluctant to express his "feelings." Not because he has too few, but, rather, because he has too many and they are difficult to manage. Like a bag of ferrets, they trouble the surface and suggest incipient commotion. When they do eventually emerge, he is voluble; not like a school board meeting in Brooklyn but more in the way of Mount Vesuvius. My brother would rather discuss digestive enzymes than his emotions and not only because he thinks a lot about digestion. So, we look around, shift on the sofa, and begin to gabble about the Knicks' playoff chances.

So much of illness is about waiting. We are generally inured to it in western civilization—we wait in lines, for phone calls, results of applications to schools or for jobs. An actor waits for a callback. A screenwriter to hear from his agent. It's annoying, but we don't dread it. Like the weather, waiting is something we tolerate. Medical waiting is different. In the world of the sick we wait for test results, to see if the treatment is working, to hear that we're cured. Thousands of dedicated rooms across the medical landscape. Waiting rooms.

My family is waiting for an idea to occur to one of us. We need something to do. Action will bring purpose and purpose will mask fear.

An outing. Shake the stink off, as Susan says. Go for a drive, or a hike in the surrounding woods. Take Allegra to a petting zoo! What better place to spend a fragrant spring day, especially when my mortality is exercising an entirely new and crushing weight? Is there anything more innocent, or gentle, anything that says yes, yes, the universe is a kind place, a loving place, a cute baby animal place, than a petting zoo? And we won't have to search for topics of conversation because we can watch Allegra commune with sheep. Children provide an excuse to embrace childish things, and everyone will be thrilled to escape the house.

Dad grabs the Yellow Pages and turns to the letter P where he quickly discovers it is not an easy thing to find a petting zoo. Relieved to have anything else to talk about, he muses that petting zoos are not a franchise-able idea like coffee or hamburgers, and thus are rare in America. They can still be found at county fairs but those cotton candy-scented jamborees are seasonal and hardly ubiquitous. What my father did locate however was a farm in Peekskill, less than an hour away, that welcomes visitors. This sounds promising. A farm, a place of growth and bounty, of life. The cocky strut of a bantam rooster will allow us to focus on something other than our collective angst.

Susan is a calm presence in the face of an uncertain future and a practical person, always partial to tasks that can be accomplished. While she packs a bag for Allegra—goldfish, diapers, baby powder—I recall childhood trips to places like the Delaware Water Gap, Howe Caverns, Palisades Amusement Park, Jones Beach, Sterling Forest, all of them emerging from a great distance, cast in the glow of a time before stress, obligations, and death, markers for innocence. Outings when my mother was alive and we were all together.

*Outings.*

Even the word has a bygone, old-timey, surrey-with-a-fringe-on-top quality. Today we will have an *outing* to a *farm.* It will be a return to the garden.

Animals have always sustained me. As a boy I esteemed dinosaurs, slobbered over dogs, was fascinated by the pigeons of New York City. Had I followed my childhood friend David into the Catholic Church there is little doubt my favorite saint would have been Francis. I marshalled a collection of stuffed animals for which I felt a deep and abiding affection and when I was old enough to have actual living, breathing pets, my joy was unbound. The menagerie included goldfish, guppies, turtles, snakes, lizards, toads, frogs, and several mice that lived in an old claw-foot bathtub on the third floor of our house until my mother found them and made me turn them loose, a rabbit, two guinea pigs, one of whom gave birth to triplets leaving us with five guinea pigs, several dogs, and a yellow parakeet. When the bird dropped from his perch I wept like a Maria Callas fan at La Scala. I was ten and that was before I became self-conscious about crying. Had I the slightest aptitude in science, I would have been a happy zoologist. Animals have always represented the *good* for me. Not in a crazy way, like the amateur naturalist who cohabitated with Alaskan grizzly bears thinking he was their friend only to discover he was their dinner. I'm not vegan, and I wear leather shoes. I am a rational animal lover. They have always provided comfort.

And comfort is what we need, the experiential equivalent of mashed potatoes and gravy. So, we pile into two cars and our little caravan proceeds to get hopelessly lost, turning what should have been a relatively short ride into the Lewis and Clark expedition because when you have cancer the universe will often decree that you are not suffering quite enough. But still, it is spring, we're out of the house, and for the time being I am alive.

After many wrong turns, we finally arrive at the farm, a ramshackle spread that hardly looks like a commercial operation, the kind of ragged, vaguely menacing property that might have a corpse or two buried under the main house, a cars-on-blocks dump, dirt and weeds. No one appears to work there but, to our surprise, several African families are milling around. Clad in Islamic mufti, the men in jubbahs, the women in burkas and headscarves. Since it would feel strange to be the only ones wandering this sinister farm, the Africans are a welcome sight.

Despite the serial-killer aesthetic of the dilapidated premises, it is still very much a farm. The air redolent of hay and manure. Goats ambling around, pigs in a pen. Skinny chickens pecking the dirt. But where are the ducks? And why do I need ducks? My mother was one of the reasons I came to love books as a child and the first book I remember her reading to me was *Make Way For Ducklings* by Robert McCloskey. Do I think the vision of a mother duck trailed by a brood of ducklings will conjure the gladdening security of my own mother's presence? Has my sudden vulnerability sent me reeling back in psychological time? Whatever the underpinnings, this farm is bereft of ducks. Instead, there are a pair of brown cows, hides drooping on unimpressive frames. The animals look like they've been beamed in from a farm in a former Soviet republic that is having trouble negotiating the transition to a free market economy.

But wait, a buffalo! Allegra's eyes widen. His immense, wooly frame is meant to be stampeding the prairie in Montana or Wyoming but here he is with his inward curving horns, mountainous shoulders, winter-thick pelt, quiescent, unmoving, in the Hudson Valley on this temperate day, the azure sky stippled with benign clouds.

We bustle toward the pen where the buffalo is pensively chewing cud. The great herds of his majestic ancestors that roamed the western plains are gone now, fallen prey to hunters and the Manifest Destiny we were taught in high school history classes, their grazing areas overgrown with towns and malls, veined with interstate highways. Unlike the other animals, all of which have confederates of their own species, there appear to be no other buffalo in the immediate area. This one is isolated, dull-eyed. It occurs to me that he might be depressed, although perhaps I am projecting. Allegra stares at this hulking apparition and I think about impermanence, how things we love disappear. How we disappear. I glance at my tiny daughter, riveted by this ghostly beast, steal a peek at my pregnant wife who is watching our daughter watching the buffalo, and contemplate the watery nature of everything. This lonely buffalo has sent me whirling toward the void. I upbraid myself for undue morbidity but then remember I have just been told I have cancer and realize a little morbidity is not inappropriate.

The farmer appears and is talking to the head of one of the Muslim families, a stocky man with a capacious beard and skin the color of obsidian. The farmer a gaunt, older white man with steel-rimmed glasses, a checked shirt, and the impassive expression of a Walker Evans subject. What are they discussing? Voices carry and we learn that Memorial Day occurs during Ramadan this year, the holiday where Muslims fast during the day and share a festive meal in the evening. It dawns on us that the friendly looking Africans are here to supervise the ritual slaughter of goats and chickens for their halal food. This is a dreadful revelation and it's all we can do to not sprint from the grim scene. One of the Muslim men selects a goat, the farmer grabs it, and he and his customers disappear into the barn. I think about the goat's straining neck pinned by the farmer's gnarled hand, the sharp blade glinting in the sepulchral light.

We have found the worst petting zoo in the world.

This was not what we came for, although if we were shopping for a resonant metaphor it would have been hard to improve upon: search for a petting zoo, find an abattoir. Far be it from me to inveigh against Muslims or their religious practices and no disparaging conclusions are to be drawn from this story. All religions have their peculiarities. Had there been a flock of Hasidim here to witness a kosher slaughter firsthand, that would be an equally salient detail. Once I saw fifty of them in Crown Heights gathered to buy live chickens, the necks of which would be swung as if they were the handles of lassos, also for a holiday celebration. But this day it is the Muslims' rural outing that coincides with our doomed endeavor and it is buzzkill of epic proportions.

We climb back into our cars and zoom off thankful Allegra

has gotten to see loveable animals and is none the wiser about the nearness of death. On the drive, we manage to not get lost. That night we drink nonalcoholic beer, eat thin-crust pizza with extra garlic from DiNardo's, and talk about nothing.

* * *

When Neil Armstrong planted the American flag on the moon, July 20th, 1969, I watched with my family on a black and white television in a motel in the desert town of Needles, California. Even at the time, I found the town's name amusing. We had driven across the country in Dad's black Cadillac Brougham with one 8-track tape: *Tommy* by the Who. By the time we reached Illinois, I had all of the lyrics committed to memory. I was thirteen years old. That summer the moon landing seemed the most hopeful accomplishment imaginable. When the astronauts landed on the lunar surface it was night-time in the California desert and the temperature was nearly a hundred degrees. Since that time it's the image of my family at night in the desert in front of the black and white television that has always been conjured by the word *needles*.

Today the long needle slips into my left wrist and a drop of blood forms on papery skin as the chemicals finally begin the journey into my veins, their toxic properties seeking to search and annihilate. My head is tilted back so I can't see the penetration of my flesh. How do junkies do it? Why would someone inject themselves with anything voluntarily? It's counterintuitive. The whole heroin experience puzzles me. You choke a vein, stab yourself with a needle, then puke and nod off? I don't get it. So: chemotherapy, with the attendant needles, is not something to which I ordinarily would have been looking forward.

But how things change! A little cancer diagnosis and all of a sudden, the needle is my best friend, boon companion, and helpmate because it carries the poison that will murder the aberrant cells and save my life. Now I love the needle, can't get enough of the needle, kiss the needle before it finds its rightful home beneath my sensitive skin. I am feeling very William Burroughs (my favorite junkie) now that Beth the Nurse has punctured a fat vein. Beth is a friendly woman with a pageboy haircut. In her early forties, she has four kids. She tells me they've had good results with this protocol. At this moment I am deeply in love with Beth.

Susan has skipped work to accompany me. Untroubled by my feelings for Beth, she remains in the waiting room and tries to get some legal business done.

A transparent bag of industrial-strength cyclophosphamide hangs on an IV pole and the clear liquid courses into my veins. Rogue cells beware—you are going down! (When thinking of cancer cells, I am careful to maintain a posture of aggressive hostility.)

I have come to the doctor's office today pumped like a pitcher playing in his first World Series, torqued, battle-ready. Give it to me, I implore. Whatever you have, I can take it. No, I can't just take it, I *want* it, okay? I fucking *want* it. This is what I'm thinking as I prepare myself for the months-long ordeal. I tell no one. Saying anything like this out loud is silly. But in my head, I am a Marine at Parris Island, *sir, yes, sir!* I am a paratrooper leaping from a plane, an astronaut blasting into space. All the images spinning through my mind are military because I am at war and I will *not* be defeated. Well, not all of them. Along with the hardened martial outlook I am now meant to embody, I will also affect the insouciance of Marcello Mastroianni in *La Dolce Vita*, because who am I kidding, I flamed out of the Boy Scouts, a pseudo-military organization for which I was blatantly unsuited. But circumstances change. The world will now see my newly granite mien threaded with saucy nonchalance.

This arduous conceptual activity is occurring while I am seated in a green vinyl-covered chair from which I will not be able to move for three hours. And I am not alone as the internal battle rages. I am in a room with five other people, none of whom are speaking to each other, all of whom are having chemotherapy, engaging with their own interior lives.

Three hours.

Three long hours absorbing poison. But I brought a book and it is not just any book. It is Martin Gilbert's "magisterial" biography of Winston Churchill. Available in paperback all over the city, but this is a big, imposing hardcover copy, a cinder block suggestive of Churchill's own impressive bulk. Ordered from Endicott Bookseller, it lies open in my lap. This book is a talisman, a Bible. I have always admired Winston Churchill in spite of his shadow side. The imposing figure, chin upturned, assured, his unflagging confidence, are inspirational. He was a sixty-five-year-old man in the political wilderness when Neville Chamberlain resigned and Great Britain turned to him and his very large cigar in 1940. He responded with some of the most remarkable oratory and copious drinking of the twentieth century. And then won a Nobel Prize. For literature. Thinking about his protean accomplishments makes me want to lie down. How does a man defeat the Germans, and then win the greatest literary prize in the world?

What follows is a passage from one of Churchill's speeches, annotated for my purposes:

(Imagine Sir Winston's stentorian cadences crackling from an old radio.)

"Even though large tracts of Europe and many old and famous states have fallen or may fall to the grip of the Gestapo *although my body is invaded by a malevolent army* and all the odious apparatus of Nazi rule, we shall not flag or fail *I am not fazed by this.* We shall fight in France *in the abdomen,* we shall fight on the seas *under the armpits* and oceans *in the groin,* we shall fight with growing confidence and growing strength in the air *the neck*, we shall defend our island *my body*, whatever the cost may be *thank god I have Writers Guild health insurance*, we shall fight on the beaches *and in the swimming pools*, we shall fight on the landing grounds *when I'm at the airport*, we shall fight on the fields *the country* and in the streets *the city*, we shall fight in the hills *Murray Hill which is the location of NYU Medical Center*; we shall never surrender, *one treatment, two treatments, three treatments*, and even if, which I do not for a moment believe, this Island *I, again,* or a large part of it were subjugated and starving *was not doing so well*, then our Empire beyond the seas *the medical profession*, armed and guarded by the British fleet *and all the powers at their considerable disposal*, would carry on the struggle, until, in God's good time, the New World, and all its power and might *they find another means*, steps forth to the rescue and the liberation of the old *and make me well*."

As you can see, it helps to personalize.

This is the reason politicians of every stripe drag out Winston Churchill. A modern Cicero, the man articulates some of our deepest and most profound aspirations. And what is deeper and more profound, as far as aspirations go, than survival? Yes, I know his legacy is complicated. His controversial tenure as Secretary of the Admiralty during WW I nearly derailed his career, his handling of India a disaster, and some of his views are problematic. In certain cases, more than problematic. Inasmuch as there is a cult that has formed around Churchill, I am a nonconformist member. But I can appreciate artistry in the films of Leni Riefenstahl, a Nazi. I've whistled a tune from a Wagner opera. The poetry of Ezra Pound continues to fascinate me despite the fact that his anti-Semitism verged on the demented. So I am willing to overlook Churchill's flaws in my current predicament. Let me assure you that I understand his shortcomings. But right now—

He is my private cheerleader.

The Germans are the cancer cells, the English and the Americans are the chemo, and together we will decimate the little Teutonic bastards just as the Nazis themselves were trounced. I read several chapters of the Churchill biography and after an hour I'm ready for a break. But I can't go anywhere since I'm hooked up to the chemo bag. In the course of my voluminous post-diagnosis reading, I discovered that visualization is a popular healing technique. It is very simple. You come up with an image that will have a positive effect on your state of mind. Then biology takes over. This is a phenomenon known as the "mind-body connection" and it is being talked about more and more by forward-thinking people in the medical community. For those who doubt the reality of the mind-body connection, I submit: a man is shown a picture of an attractive naked woman. He gets an erection. Case closed.

It's actually a little more complicated than that.

But not much.

I close my eyes and let a movie unspool.

I am on a beach. The beach, white sand and tropical, is invaded by cancerous gremlins that run around chattering madly, drinking rum, smashing into each other, scratching, clawing, humping, humping, humping. A large wave appears on the azure horizon. As the wave rolls toward the shore, it gains in size and force, building, growing, you can hear it now, louder, *LOUDER*. By the time it smashes into the beach, it is overwhelming. The gremlins? Gasping! Choking! Drowning! Many die. Another wave appears, more powerful than the first. The remaining gremlins, already soaked and decimated, are cringing. It crashes onto them and carries their pitiful remnants out to the sea, dead, dead, dead, and vanquished forever.

I am relaxed when this is over.

This feeling of being relaxed is pleasurable, novel even. I

have not been relaxed much lately and I want to be more relaxed. How can this be achieved?

When the cyclophosphamide has drained out of its bag, Beth reloads with Fludarabine.

Drip, drip, drip.

I continue to visualize the internal battle. More gremlins, more waves.

Several hours later I am done. Beth gives me Compazine to combat the nausea which, I have been informed, will be arriving on the evening train. Susan greets me in the waiting room and asks how I'm feeling. Terrific, I tell her, and try to manufacture a smile. Her green eyes flash with hope. I place my hand on her expanding belly.

That night I feel all right although I don't sleep well. I go for treatment the next day, and the next. By the time I have spent the better part of three days on the receiving end of the chemo drugs, I am having trouble pretending to feel good. I am flagging and, despite the Compazine, nauseous. I'm not throwing up, but if I were, perhaps I would feel better. By the end of the fourth day I am weak and logy. I am constipated. No one told me having chemo would be like swallowing glue. To complete the voiding picture, I am having trouble urinating. And I have no appetite. All I want to do it lie down and suck ice cubes.

I hang around the apartment and let the chemicals marinate. When I am traveling back and forth to the hospital for the treatment I am struck by how normal everyone appears. That they carry their invisible burdens and afflictions I'm well aware, but the people I encounter on the subway all seem exceedingly unperturbed in my deeply subjective point of view. Even the ones who don't look healthy are probably a lot healthier than I am. In my predicament, I am the other, the science experiment.

A few days later I receive the results of the bone aspiration.

The radiologist who examines the film looks for the cancer cells to spread to the liver, the spleen, or the marrow. It is in none of these places and this is the first bit of good news we've received. I allow myself a dollop of optimism. Still, I long for the time when Needles came with a capital "N" and meant the California desert and my family and the moon landing.

# PART 3
## MUDDLING THROUGH

The first time the two of us talk about meditation we are in our dining room overlooking Amsterdam Avenue. It is early evening and the sky is bruised purple. Susan has cooked a macrobiotic dinner that I am desperately trying to enjoy. Tofu and an unidentifiable vegetable she claims is okra. Hard to know since I don't think I've ever seen okra. It feels penitential, more like a punishment than a meal, but if this is what getting well takes, I am on board. Susan was raised in a place where the three food groups consist of meat, something white, and dessert. Although her own palate is now considerably more refined, she is still a lover of steaks, chops, ribs. And she salts most things. Cooking this new way is a sacrifice, both cultural and culinary. She is cheerful about this fresh dietary world, excited to be able to help. Allegra is seated in her high chair at the table, smearing baby food around her mouth. Somehow, I know her dinner is tastier than the swill I am attempting to consume.

Where has our normal food gone? It has all been thrown out by Susan in a frenzy of purification. The presence of disease has understandably ratcheted up her anxiety and this purging of the kitchen cabinets is the immediate result. I gaze longingly at a blue box of Ronzoni spaghetti peeking out of the garbage. Susan offers a reproachful look. There will be no white flour pasta for me. She places what is meant to be a consoling hand on my shoulder. I can feel her edginess, almost as if it is being transferred to me. How am I supposed to be able to relax if she is thrumming?

Forlornly, I spear a cube of tofu, place it in my mouth, and ask, "What do you think about meditation?"

She chews her rubbery tofu, trying not to grimace at the taste. Her carnivorous Michigan background does not embrace the East, and by East, I am not referring to New York but, rather, the part of the world home to the great contemplative traditions. Presbyterians as a rule are not a group that sits on cushions and meditates. They are more traditionally found on sofas knitting or watching college football on TV. This has the potential to be a major step.

"Meditation?" Attempting to not sound surprised but her voice goes up an octave. "Really?"

"We should try it once."

"What's that going to do?"

"Calm you down, for one thing."

"I'm not calm?"

I lift an eyebrow. Her inner storm is leaking. But meditation? How can she possibly do that? She is a talker, an arguer, a person whose first response to being told to do anything is to ask why. Enforced quiescence is less appealing than okra.

"I did a little investigating and they have weekly classes at the Zen Center. I want us to go."

She regards me suspiciously. The *Zen Center*? Susan attended the Paw Paw Presbyterian Church where she sang in the choir. She collects Christmas ornaments. Now she's supposed to go to the Zen Center? In any marriage, it's important to try new things. I remind her that she once enrolled us in a ballroom dancing class. Other people wrap themselves in cellophane, I remember thinking, so who was I to judge? We went one time and felt goofy, although we enjoyed fooling around together, attempting the steps, tripping, laughing. She reminds me that the two of us generally shy away from group activities. She agrees that meditation might be worth exploring if for no other reason than to tame the twin hurricanes between our ears.

She asks, "What are you supposed to think about while you're meditating?"

"I have no idea."

"Do you get a mantra?"

"I think that's TM. This is Zen. Anyway, how hard can it be?"

The truth is, I don't particularly want to meditate either. While I am normally comfortable living in my own head, now the idea of being alone with my thoughts with nothing to distract me is as appealing as a weekend in Yemen. Meditation in this context is tofu-like, more of a punishment than anything else.

*You're vulnerable and terrified? Sit with those thoughts.*

And yet. Perhaps it will help us be—*Zen.*

"I can't think about nothing," she says. Well, that's two of us. But Susan is conscious that this is important to me and if I want to do it, then she has to at least try.

Meditation has never been something to which I've gravitated. I wish this were not so since I would be a better person if it were, a person less in need of meditation. My brother has been meditating seriously since college. He is either far more relaxed than I, or extremely good at faking it. When he spent time in California years earlier he became a practitioner of Siddha Yoga and a disciple of its Bollywood-pretty leader, Swami Chidvilasananda, aka Gurumayi. The practitioners' devotion to her is total and when my brother talks about the guru his eyes glow. She would be a leading candidate were anyone to attempt to produce a guru cheesecake calendar. But her appeal goes beyond this.

Years earlier, at a family wedding, Drew and I met a cousin of a cousin who was a follower of someone known as the Maharaji, billed as the Sixteen-year-old Perfect Master. This cousin of a cousin banged on rapturously about how he had "heard the music and tasted the nectar." My brother and

I looked at each other like this guy had beamed in from some other planet, one where the Jews had clearly lost their minds. How can it be then, that my sibling has his very own guru? Now he listens to his guru's tapes; there is a picture of her in his car. He traveled to Ganeshpuri, India, to learn the techniques at the bubbling font. In high school he was captain of the basketball team, epicenter of a group of friends, smoked weed, danced to the Grateful Dead, checked all suburban white-boy boxes. But there was also an aggressive side that he has taken great pains to tame. Once, while playing a game of family doubles on a local tennis court, we found ourselves on opposite sides of the net, at close range. When the ball came to him, he did not hold back and smashed it at me with a velocity that verged on the assaultive. Not at my feet or in a way that I would have had to reach in order to return it, no. Like a bullet directed at my upper body. No rule breaking was involved but it was startlingly aggressive, as if he were enacting a primal instinct. That long-ago afternoon, the idea that this person who had just tried to murder me with a tennis ball would one day live in an ashram was risible. Then in college: change. He adopted vegetarianism, began meditating, studied astrology, numerology, different non-Western modes of thought and being. He had never evinced the slightest interest in this rodeo and now he was saddling up. On a humorless path whose destination I couldn't discern, and with the zeal of the newly converted, for a time he became inscrutable.

Along with rabbis, priests, and imams I have always been suspicious of gurus who imply they have achieved earthly perfection. While this is impossible, it is a shuck and jive that has nonetheless been around for millennia. Then came my brother's four years in an ashram, meditating for endless hours, scarfing vegetarian food, perfecting his current incarnation. My parents were beside themselves. My mother reacted as if he

had become a bank robber. Dad wanted to have the Siddha
Yoga finances investigated. But Drew just meditated and
chanted and exuded sanguinity. To earn money, he produced
college recruiting videos, even hired me to write one. He convinced the people who ran the ashram to allow him to have a
television in his room so he could watch basketball. It wasn't
as if he wanted to live in a cave. In a cave, you can't get cable.
My brother has joined our father in the advertising business
now, but he carries the ashram with him.

Unlike the side of my brother that wanted cable, his spiritual turn was never something with which I could connect. I
have always been profoundly of the world. The kind of meditation he practiced seemed druglike to me. I had never done
TM when that was popular. The whole idea behind meditation
was utterly alien and having my only sibling fall under the sway
of a guru, however pulchritudinous, did nothing to help my
attitude. It is easy to maintain this point of view in America
because many people will reinforce it. We do not live in a meditative culture. The introspective individual is run over by the
shotgun-wielding yahoo in a pickup truck with a credit card
between his teeth on his way to a Presidents' Day sale. America
is about getting and spending and woe to him who takes time
out—other than Sunday morning with Jesus—for a few quiet
moments. Mainstream spirituality in America is result-ori-
ented. People pray for health, or wealth, or their children, or
parents, or pets, or new shoes, making requests, calling a help
line, dial-a-deity. I do not exclude myself from this cohort of
pushy spirituality, since in the last few days I have indulged in
my own pathetic attempt at prayer.

As a people, Americans are often heard giving thanks to
God. And the next thing out of our mouths is *Now that I have
your attention, God/Jesus/divine-being-of-your-choice, there's
one more thing—*

Even yoga, the venerable Hindu version of physical fitness,

undergoes a shift in America. A yogi in India twists himself into a contemplative pretzel and lowers his body temperature with his mind, stillness and quietude emulating that of a frozen dinner, while his American cousin participates in so-called "power yoga." This Western iteration of yoga practice is a stunning marriage of two antithetical traditions: people leaping around, heart rates pumping at remarkable levels, limbs flying for an hour before placing their hands together, drenched in sweat, exhausted, bowing their heads and saying *Namaste.*

My friend Andy's brother joined an Eastern religious order and changed his name from Jeffrey to Akasha. Andy called him Akasha Varnishkes, after the famous Eastern European carbohydrate. That always struck me as the correct response to this kind of conversion. When the Beatles flitted to India to meditate with the Maharishi Mahesh Yogi, I was fascinated by their choice, but utterly uninterested in exploring it. The only detail I recall about their entire adventure is that Ringo brought a suitcase full of peanut butter so he wouldn't get dysentery, and the Maharishi allegedly tried to seduce someone's girlfriend which turns out to be a pretty common guru perk. When George remained the only true believer and incorporated Indian influences in his music, I enjoyed the songs but, to be honest, not as much as his other stuff. Who will argue that "Within You and Without You" gives greater pleasure than "Here Comes the Sun"? For years, when I would walk down the street in Manhattan and see the Hare Krishnas capering in their orange robes, clanging their finger cymbals and generally making merry, I would think: *look at those chumps.* The Hare Krishna style manual called for them to shave their heads but leave one long lock extruding from the top. They believe one of their many gods is going to reach down from Heaven, grab on to this, and yank them skyward. I thought: What kind of simpleton believes this? How do they expect anyone to take them seriously? And their chanting was distinguished largely by its capacity to annoy. I'm not proud of this reaction. It is judgmental and small-minded. These are simply people who held no brief for the spiritual traditions of the West and searched for succor in more exotic quarters. Who am I, someone with no spiritual life, to cast aspersions? Particularly now that I think a spiritual life might be something from which I can benefit.

The following evening, Susan and I arrive at the Zen Center on East 67th Street. It's on the second floor of an unremarkable townhouse. We are gathered with ten other initiates and given a talk by a robed white guy named Steve who informs us he is a *roshi*, or priest. The room is oblong, about forty feet by fifteen feet. The walls are painted white, the floor covered with tan industrial carpet. The lights are dim. I listen intently as he discourses on the basic techniques and positions. Briefly, here they are: you sit on a cushion with your legs crossed and think about nothing. This turns out to be far more difficult than it sounds.

There is a type of personality that reacts to stress with laughter and occasionally I have fallen into that category. For the duration of Roshi Steve's talk, I don't make eye contact with Susan because I am afraid I might start laughing and I know that once that begins it may not stop in a timely or dignified manner. I don't want to laugh now because it would be disrespectful to our instructor. Frankly, laughter would be a gift, sustaining and curative, and it would be the first time I laughed in days. But it would not be appropriate (my mother's influence) so I do not look at Susan who is able to send me into paroxysms of hilarity with a raised eyebrow.

Roshi Steve produces a metal bowl and a stick. He tells us to get in a single file line for a walking meditation. It strikes me as a good compromise since moving at least gives you something to think about while you're meditating that doesn't count as actual thought—don't step on the guy in front of me, I hope that person behind me doesn't step on my heel, when is this going to be over?

Roshi Steve whacks the bowl with his stick, there's a humming sound, and we start to move. We pad quietly around the room several times. I breathe deeply but when I try to think about nothing, I fail. I'm thinking I want to be somewhere else, like a Knicks game. I'm thinking I'd like to eat a delicious cut of ribeye steak cooked medium rare. I'm thinking I wouldn't be in the New York Zen Center walking in circles with a bunch of strangers if I were healthy.

Roshi Steve strikes the bowl again—the high, tuning fork hum—and we stop walking. He then asks us to sit in a row facing the wall. We park ourselves on meditation cushions which we learn are called zafus. I settle in, relax my shoulders, straighten my back, and begin:

*How am I supposed to stop thinking? I can't stop thinking. I think every second I'm awake and if my dreams are any indication, I'm thinking when I'm asleep, mostly thoughts of fear and consternation but that's a kind of thinking, isn't it? My leg is starting to hurt. When I wake up, I think: Should I get out of bed, or lie here for a few more minutes? Then I get up and it's Do I shower before or after I eat breakfast? Then it's Cereal or toast? Then it's Sneakers or shoes? I read the paper and it's Do I like the Mayor today; do I like the President? And how did that guy I went to film school with get a movie he wrote produced? He never seemed that talented. Am I going to make it to the gym or if I have a productive morning at my desk can I see a movie in the afternoon? What's playing? Should I see the movie written by the guy I know from film school? By 8:00 A.M. my head is already like Grand Central Station at rush hour before a holiday. My nose itches. How can I stop thinking if my nose is itching? I have an itchy nose. Does that even qualify as a thought? I*

*can't scratch it because someone will see me move and think
I can't sit still. I am uncomfortable with the thought of these
people judging me. Who are they to judge me? I know they're
here to learn meditation but why are they really here? I don't
want to observe my thoughts. My thoughts follow each other
in such rapid succession I could sprain my neck watching
them. My leg really hurts now. Meditation is not for someone
like me. But Zoloft! With Zoloft, at least you don't have to
look into every little nook and cranny in your head. Sitting
with Roshi White Man Steve and a bunch of strangers on
cushions cannot possibly be what I need. I like Keith
Richards. He probably doesn't meditate although I can't be
certain. Who thought of yogurt? What was the name of that
restaurant on Long Island, the shack near the beach where I
had that amazing sandwich when I was ten years old? I think
it was called Gene's—or maybe it was Jerry's—something
with a G or a J—how long have I been sitting here? If I look
at my watch will anyone notice? That leg is killing me—*

And then the first minute ended.

My mind alternately races and slows. At one point, I fight the
urge to laugh but it passes quickly. The hysteria I fear does not
materialize. To go with the leg pain, I now have some back pain.

What's that? Movement!

I sense someone behind me bolt toward the door, an
escapee, Zen jailbreak! They can't take it anymore. I feel
momentarily superior then glance toward Susan to catch her
eye. But her zafu is empty. I swing my head around and look
toward the door just in time to see her run out of the room. It
was she! My pregnant wife, my companion in all things new,
the woman whom I dragged to this place, is sprinting out of
the room. I surmise she is not enjoying being alone with her
thoughts, quite understandably given what they must be.

I continue to meditate. It takes a Herculean effort to keep

my hands held loosely in my lap. Most shocking to me is my ability to sit there the entire time.

After half an hour Steve strikes the bowl again to end the meditation. He leads us in a chant and then we are served green tea. Susan sidles up smiling and informs me she is more relaxed now that she has stopped meditating. We are told this is the time to ask questions. A young woman wants to know whether it is acceptable to meditate lying down. Steve informs her that Zen meditation requires that the practitioner be seated on the ground. If pain occurs, we're supposed to sit through it. Meditation, apparently, is about endurance. It's about suffering. This is something I can understand.

Susan and I are walking home.

"Why did you run out of the room?"

She looks at me like I'm crazy. "I can't sit on a cushion and think about nothing." It's a balmy evening and I'm feeling more relaxed now that we've left the Zen Center. Susan quietly explains that on top of continuing to work full time, she has been so busy trying to fix our life that feelings about being pregnant while already caring for a toddler and a husband with cancer that can get pushed aside in the course of an average day came rushing back while she was planted on a zafu. I see her point. We stop at a red light when we hit Lexington Avenue. I take her hand. Neither of us say anything when we cross the street.

I ask Susan if she's going to keep meditating.

"You saw me in there."

"What do you mean?"

"I nearly ran out of the building." She laughs, shakes her head at the memory. Then we're both laughing. The two of us are usually up for experience and like the ballroom dancing class we once signed up for, it seemed a good idea at the time. "I can't meditate," Susan concludes. "You should do it, though."

\* \* \*

I feel like bad weather and my sleep is wrecked. Sores in my mouth and strange pains in my legs. After two cycles of chemotherapy I'm trying to remain optimistic while losing weight I don't want to be losing since I'm already skinny. I consider my hair. Buddha is bald. This is what is going through my mind as I close my eyes and try to achieve a meditative state, a difficult task as the downtown train barrels beneath Manhattan. And what makes it harder is that I can't stop thinking about baldness. I am riding the subway to the East Village running my hands through my hair. Thinning a little on the crown, but not noticeably. A young Hispanic couple sits across from me holding hands, vibrant with health, their lives in front of them. She: gold hoop earrings, thick, dark hair pulled back in a ponytail that glistens in the fluorescent subway light. He: sweatshirt with a Mets logo, running shoes. His hair is short and full. They both have great hair. This is not a thought that would have occurred a few weeks ago.

The heroes of my teenage years, rock stars mostly (the ones who were not basketball players), all had rebellious hair and I wanted to emulate them. Had I been given free rein my hair would have cascaded down my back and to my waist. But free rein was not given and I lived haircut to haircut, willing my locks over my ears and down my neck. My hair length was a never-ending battle with my mother who, for reasons I still do not understand, particularly given her fondness for Joan Baez albums and playing folk guitar, despised long hair on boys. She used to say, "If your hair gets any longer we're going to have to buy you a violin." It was a remarkably anachronistic cultural reference since violinists were not remotely on my radar. She would also sing "Barney Google, with the googly-googly eyes . . . " a 1930s ditty, so staying current was not a theme.

I get off the train at Astor Place, bound up the subway stairs, and into a blast of early summer heat. I'm ready. Astor Place Haircutters is across the street. A subterranean refuge entered by descending a concrete stairwell. Large and airy, the salon is crowded with punky hipsters having their identities shaped by the overworked staff. There I am in the mirror, a final image of what will soon be the person I used to look like.

The stylist is a stout young woman in a black dress. Red lipstick, ghostly skin, hair chopped short and dyed pink. Clunky, thick-soled shoes; black, horn-rimmed glasses. How much do you want me to take off, she asks. All of it, I say. She revs the electric clipper, leans in. Off it comes on the left side, off on the right. There's a Mohawk until the top is sheared. My hair is gone now. This is not to affect a monkish look, to announce my solidarity with my brothers from the east, the Buddhist masters. I shave my head because I don't want to find hair on my pillow, in my drain. I don't want to lose my hair. Losing your hair to chemotherapy is a show of weakness to me, one that displays a lack of control (never mind that I can't control anything at this point).

Shaving my head, conversely, is an assertion of power. A complement to my soldierly approach. It will make me look macho, I tell myself, not like some weedy cancer patient.

I take a last look at my new identity and decide to give mirrors a rest for a while.

When I get back to the apartment, I try to meditate.

It does not escape me that with my newly shorn head and nascent exploration of contemplative practice I am closer to that raucous saffron mob of sidewalk finger cymbalists than ever before. This makes me laugh.

\* \* \*

There are people who love talk therapy. Whether Freudian,

Jungian, or the many contemporary iterations of this venerable treatment protocol, great swaths of humanity have benefitted from downloading their problems into the ear of a sympathetic professional. I am not one of them. Therapy is not something I usually think about and this is not because I haven't tried to parse my troubles with a psychologist. I'm just terrible at it. It is late in the day and Susan and I are taking a pre-dinner constitutional on West 83rd Street. We're heading toward Central Park, pushing Allegra in her carriage. In the gloaming, the air is warm and the summer humidity has not arrived. It is a flawless Manhattan moment. People on the sidewalk, flowing home from work, going out for the evening. To me their lives look perfect. Our daughter takes it all in. She is babbling but not making a lot of sense since she can't really talk.

My veins are shimmering with napalm. The third course of chemo.

We hit Central Park West and head south, past the Museum of Natural History. As a child I was particularly fascinated by the panoramas of Early Man. Now, I consider whether Early Men had any knowledge of death or was their perception like that of, say, a dog or a horse? There is a permanence to the Museum of Natural History that I take comfort in. Susan breaks into my thoughts and says, "I learned about this therapist today."

"Oh, yeah?" My attention has been drawn by a pizza place on Columbus Avenue. I want to eat pizza for dinner but pizza is now my enemy.

"This guy is supposed to be gifted. He's a serious healer." She's heard that he possesses unseen reservoirs of empathy, insight, and compassion. Susan is a believer in the efficacy of therapy. A beneficiary of several years of it herself, a leitmotif of our relationship is her urging its benefits on me personally and on us in couples counseling.

"He sounds great," I say, thinking of pepperoni. I'm not

interested, but don't want to shut Susan down. "What else can you tell me about him?"

"Well," she says "He's a quadriplegic."

"A *quadriplegic!*" I nearly shout.

"What's wrong with that?"

"There's nothing *wrong* with it, per se."

"So what's the problem?"

"How am I supposed to complain to a quadriplegic?" I ask, baffled. "That's got to be the whole basis of his practice. 'Your wife left you?'" I say, pretending to be the quadriplegic therapist. "'Oooo, too baaaddd. At least you can run after her, you whiny little shit! I'm a quadriplegic!'"

Susan laughs but I can tell she is disappointed with my reaction. It is clear this will not work since I am already feeling guilty without having even met the man. "Don't give up on the idea of therapy," she implores.

"I won't," I say. "As long as the mental health professional is a functioning biped."

Susan snorts, but I know she really wants me to talk to a therapist.

It needs to be pointed out, at the risk of offending the differently-abled, that were I not hosting a house party for a surfeit of mutating cells a quadriplegic therapist would be a non-issue. But as it is, I believe my own powers of empathy will compromise the therapy process. I would want to take care of him. That is not the idea.

Most people I know have, at one time or another, been in some kind of therapy. On the Upper West Side of Manhattan, ground zero for the therapeutic community, it is the zeitgeist, like baseball in Cooperstown, the quality that suffuses a place with meaning. Once, twice, or even five times a week for some analysands, the citizenry puts their work down and traipses to an office where a nonjudgmental professional with several letters after her name listens to them grouse for an hour, sometimes commenting, mostly absorbing the vexatious words without responding. This technique, the "talking cure," seems mostly palliative in effect. People yammer until they are tired of hearing what they have to say, after which they connect the dots and, it is hoped, are better able to function.

Only recently, I had reluctantly acceded to the therapeutic imperative and entered couples counseling with Susan. Our marriage was solid but there were certain family of origin issues that we thought could be better resolved with an impartial referee. Seated in the office, we examined our relationship with a microscope. Apparently, the two of us needed to listen more and hector less, not exactly a stunningly original insight but nonetheless good advice for most couples. We went for three sessions and then I was diagnosed with lymphoma. I informed Susan that I was done with couples counseling since it was obvious that therapy causes cancer. She took this good-naturedly.

In my view, I have already failed at therapy.

But now the emotional playing field has changed and I am no longer so fancy free.

Susan, Allegra and I pass Gray's Papaya. The usual suspects are wolfing down hot dogs, tubes of meat by-product which, in my larval state of enlightenment, I now realize are nothing more than insidious, if tasty, delivery systems for animal growth hormones and cancer-causing nitrites. Don't those people shoving carcinogenic grease pockets down their throats know they're killing themselves? Don't they care? I want to run in there and yell at them to save themselves before it is too late, to change their lives and embrace health, clean living, and enlightenment.

I resist the impulse.

Dr. Barbuto is in his forties with the bushy mustache of a vaudevillian. I am greatly relieved when he rises to greet me.

No wheelchair with a breath controller. It is obvious he can walk so I feel free to hit him with both barrels. But once in his nurturing, therapeutic presence, my survival instinct takes over, a need that braids machismo and pride and requires that no one witness me suffering, including anyone who has been retained to do precisely that.

I sit across from him in a chair and feel like I am performing the role of someone talking to a therapist. Since my diagnosis, I have gone from fear, to sadness, to anger, to Churchillian resolve. I have learned that while I am a person who can be thrown off-kilter by small things, when it comes to big ones I am consistently functional. When Dr. Barbuto asks me how I am feeling, the following review occurs in a blink: I obsess about my bowel movements. Hard, soft, pellet-like, I read them like tea leaves for clues to my well-being. I get dizzy sometimes when I stand up. I have a tingling sensation in my thigh. I wonder if I'll ever feel like myself again or is this what it means to feel like myself now. Will I be prey to a series of small ailments that are going to grow larger and eventually engulf me? The other night, this thought—tingling, numbness—I have multiple sclerosis. I'm a hypochondriac now. Can you have cancer and be a hypochondriac or do they cancel each other out? I think about time, how quickly it moves, how the days and weeks hurtle by faster and faster. Only man understands time. This knowledge is an immeasurable burden, the price of biting the apple in the Garden. Adam and Eve recognizing their nakedness makes the story about sex. But who cares about sex? The devastating piece of knowledge, the one that undergirds everything, the one that begets our deepest fears is that of time, tick, tick, tick, one year, five years, ten years, nothing is enough. My kids are going to grow up without a father which almost bothers me more than the thought of my own death. I feel like this illness has increased my perceptions to an almost unbearable degree.

But I do not *say* any of that.

Here is what I say: "Under the circumstances, fine."

"Can you work?"

"I took two days off when I found out I was sick and then I went back to my desk."

"Are you eating?"

"Yes."

"Any problems sleeping?"

"I take a pill."

No emotions, no histrionics. It turns out that when it comes to compartmentalization, I have heretofore undiscovered skills. After determining that I can work, sleep, and eat without too much trouble, he tells me he anticipates I will have coping difficulties in the future and I should keep seeing him since I obviously need to be in therapy. Not wanting to hurt his feelings, another appointment is scheduled.

I cancel it a few days later.

My experience with Dr. Barbuto puzzles me because, like him, I think I should be falling apart. The fact that I am not seems somehow wrong. Am I too good at compartmentalizing? Is that not my part in the narrative, to be the tragic victim, to caterwaul, rail at the fates? Wouldn't it feel good to just let go and disintegrate? Turns out I am not good at being a victim. I was trying, though. I had gone to see the therapist, hadn't I? In *Four Quartets,* the ever-quotable T.S. Eliot writes that humankind cannot bear too much reality. Am I one of the people he was referring to? Am *I* delusional?

Distrustful of my own reaction, I think, perhaps it is Dr. Barbuto's inability to tease out my suffering that is the problem. Everyone says I will benefit from therapy, so why not try again? Dutifully, I make another appointment, this one with Dr. Wyczinsky, a tall, sober woman with an office in a high rise. After a repeat of the conversation with Dr. Barbuto, she informs me, to my relief, that I am doing fine under the circumstances but if there's a problem in the future, she will be glad to help.

I wonder why it is unnecessary to unload on these therapists and then it occurs to me—not only am I functional in my day to day life, but I am so affronted by what has occurred, so put out, that my internal response has slid from the initial astonishment and sorrow all the way to *aggression*, not toward the therapists—both of whom I liked—but within my own mind. I can win this battle, and the less moaning the better.

Straighten the spine, throw back the shoulders. And as Dad would say, march forth.

That night, we eat dinner at home. Since Susan has made the improvement of my diet a personal crusade, it is some kind of macrobiotic slop that she is cooking for the first time as an experiment. Although it tastes like cement I consume it wondering why, if macrobiotic food is so healthy, does everyone I've ever met who is on a macrobiotic diet look so unwell? Then Susan hands me a small brown bottle.

"What's this?"

"Shark cartilage."

If Susan gave me a bottle containing bison hoof I would not blink. What is shark cartilage supposed to do, I wonder?

"It's an alternative cancer treatment," she says.

That's good enough for me. Immediately, I open the bottle and pop one in my mouth. I have no idea how it's supposed to work, what it does, or if it's anything other than a particularly colorful folk remedy. But none of that matters. At this point, I am willing to try anything.

Shark cartilage? At least it's not therapy.

\* \* \*

My friend Max and I are at the Broadway Deli in the early

afternoon. Max is drinking coffee. I am drinking herbal tea since I no longer allow myself caffeine. I am a man with a shaved head sipping herbal tea because coffee is part of a conspiracy to kill me. As for the food on the menu, I'm not interested. The anti-nausea drugs have been working so at least I'm not puking. I have also been trying to meditate. My skill level is low but I am able to spend several minutes sitting in complete silence while not freaking out. Max and I met through our mutual friend Leonard, to whom I have turned in the past for emotional support and jokes. Today Leonard is doing field research for a book he is co-writing with his wife about spiritual places in metropolitan New York (not a joke). His easygoing presence is missed because Max is very intense. His whole being is declarative.

"There was a growth on my neck and I went to see a doctor," Max is saying. "The doctor told me it was cancer. But I didn't want chemotherapy, okay? So I went to see this man in Chinatown and he cured me. The tumor shrunk, and then it went away. This guy can cure your lymphoma."

This guy can cure my lymphoma? Could it be possible? Was there some obscure Asian healer hidden away in the warrens of lower Manhattan, ignored by the mainstream medical profession, practicing his craft in obscurity and poverty, who could, contravening all traditional medical pronouncements, *cure* me?

Most of my friends, when they heard I had lymphoma, wanted to know if they could do anything. I appreciated the question, but since they could not cure cancer, the answer was always no. Max, exponent of all things Eastern (he is thrilled that I have converted to meditation, however uneasily, or temporarily), who jokingly refers to himself as Sri Maximus Doodle, a satirical play on the name of Sri Chinmoy, a famous guru, fits into another category. Max is unusual among my crowd in that he presents as a genuine tough guy. And not just a tough guy but a tough Jew, something of which he is inordinately proud. Most of my friends grew up in the suburbs; college-educated, enviable careers, men and women who avoid bar fights. Max, on the other hand, is from Newark and if there is an American town less privileged than that, I have yet to hear about it. He is a boxer with the busted nose to prove it. Max is coy about details but alludes to crime both petty and not-so-petty and a serious relationship with a porn actress. He is also an author. As a young man, he published a novel that boasted a blurb from a celebrated Beat writer. Max is a lot like Jean Genet, minus the gay sex. Had he been a Frenchman during World War II he would have been in the underground and relished the killing of Nazis. More than relishing killing them, he would have relished describing how he did it in long monologues. I am a little surprised he is telling me that Chinese herbs cured him. He seems like the kind of guy who would simply take a hard look at whatever disease had the temerity to set up shop in his body and then beat it into submission with his callused fists.

I am happy to take him up on his offer.

The next day we meet at his pre-gentrification Hell's Kitchen apartment which with its ziggurat of dirty dishes, pine and cinder-block bookshelves sagging under the weight of endless tattered paperbacks, and batik-draped furniture looks like it could double as a set from the movie version of any Kerouac novel. From there we take the subway downtown. On Elizabeth Street we find the herbal shop of Dr. Shen nestled between two Chinese restaurants with glazed ducks hanging in the windows. Long, narrow, and dark, it looks as if it has been moved piece by piece from its original location in the Forbidden City and painstakingly reconstructed in lower Manhattan. As for Dr. Shen, so does he. Ancient and gaunt, his thick glasses magnify tired, rheumy eyes. I have no idea whether he is a doctor in the western sense, a fellow who has gone to a medical school and is conversant with what we think of as medicine, or whether he is a folk healer, a sprite that extracts remedies from roots and berries. I really don't care. It wouldn't matter to me if he had a bone through his nose. Dr. Shen takes us to a small examination room in the back of the shop. At his request I remove my shirt.

"You look pale," he says.

I wonder if this was because he is accustomed to seeing Chinese people.

Max speaks bluntly to Dr. Shen: "My friend has lymphoma. Can you cure that?"

Dr. Shen leans in and examines me more closely. My heart freezes. Is he going to say yes, no problem, of course?

What he says is this: "I no can cure lymphoma."

*I no can cure lymphoma?*

What kind of shit is that?

The exalted Dr. Shen, the Wizard of Elizabeth Street, has failed to live up to his billing and for a moment, Max, ever voluble, is stupefied. He nods mutely and does not meet my disappointed glance. I have allowed magical thinking to intrude. The idea that a Chinese wizard held the key to my wellness and would cure me with some enchanted elixir is powerful juju.

I land back on earth with a frame-shaking thud. Despite my newfound, meditation-induced calm, I feel disappointment mixing with hostility. But the rising bile passes momentarily and I regain my emotional equilibrium, at least what passes for emotional equilibrium these days which basically means I can control the impulse to run down the sidewalk waving my arms and screaming.

Dr. Shen says he will prescribe a tea to boost my immune system. Anger and fear rear up again. I came down here desperately hoping that this obscure Asian magus could confound the Western know-it-alls and all he can prescribe is tea? Tea! If I wanted *tea*, I could have gone to Tung Sing Hunan on Columbus Avenue, where they serve it by the bucket.

I wrestle with the snarky voice in my head, the one saying: *You come to this neighborhood when you want Kung Pao Chicken, you fool, not a cure for a disease.*

Then the anger at Dr. Shen shifts again and I realize I'm angry at myself. For grasping at straws, for being ill. But anger, as some people must learn again and again, is not a helpful stance.

I take a deep breath.

Perhaps he can't cure me, but neither can the doctors at NYU or Memorial Sloan-Kettering. My immune system, however, will get a boost. The day will not be wasted. I have a new straw to grasp.

Here is my thinking: the chemotherapy will get rid of the cancer. My immune system will be strengthened. The cancer will not come back because I will have repaired my immune system. I came to Chinatown hoping to hear old Dr. Shen say *yes of course I can cure you* and my disappointment at not hearing those words continues to resonate. But I am taking the long view and something good, however small, will come from this encounter.

Dr. Shen takes us to the front of the shop where two of his young assistants arrange seven placemats on the glass counter. From the countless wooden drawers on the wall behind them they remove a selection of mysterious natural remedies and mix them into seven different piles. These are comprised of what appear to be twigs, dried leaves, and bark. It all looks revolting but that hardly matters. Each is placed in a brown paper lunch bag. Dr. Shen explains that one bag is to work for two days. He tells me to put half the contents of a bag into five cups of water then boil it down to one cup which I should then drink. On the second day I am supposed to place the remaining contents of the bag into three cups of water and boil it down to one cup before drinking. Hundreds of millions of people in China believe this works.

Can they all be wrong?

That night I follow Dr. Shen's instructions and place half the contents of one bag in five cups of water. As it boils down to its essence, an acrid scent fills the apartment. I think of the witches in *Macbeth* hovering over the bubbling cauldron. The brew looks like something you would use to clean an axle. Susan and Allegra are repulsed when they smell it. After about half an hour I am staring down a cup of viscous, horrible-smelling swampish excrescence. But I need to boost my immune system, so drink up! I manage to ingest the stuff, fighting the gag reflex, and drain the entire contents of the cup. I follow this procedure for the next nine nights and it does not get easier or more palatable. I have no idea whether it actually *does* anything, but I act on the notion that anything that is supposed to help will have some positive effect even if it is only psychological. And even if the effect is primarily psychological, that in itself is no small thing. A big part of battling illness is maintaining a positive state of mind, believing you are doing whatever is within your power to act against what has laid you low. A lot of people believe this is "woo-woo" and dismiss it but here's the theory: for healing to effectively occur the body can't be in a state of stress. Negative thoughts are stressful. Still too "woo-woo"? If there is a venerable healing tradition that requires the contents of some herbal magician's toxic bag of tricks, I will be the one saying "Abracadabra."

Sri Maximus Doodle is disappointed that Dr. Shen did not live up to his billing as a world class healer and wants to do more to help me. Along with being a meditation devotee and a consumer of horrible-smelling Chinese herbs, Max is a practitioner of the martial art known as qigong, more popularly known simply as tai chi. Tai chi is based on the Chinese theory of chi, or loosely, life force. The theory goes something like this: every human has chi, it bounds around the body literally animating us. Chi travels on meridians that run horizontally and vertically. All illnesses, its enthusiasts believe, result from a blockage of the sick person's chi. Tai chi is intended to open the meridians and allow for maximum flow of chi. Clearly, my chi could use some help. It has bogged down, stopped running.

Undaunted by the Chinese herb experience, I agree to accompany Max to the lair of his teacher, Master Chu. Master Chu's dojo is located on the second floor of a run-down building in the West Forties. Up a dark flight of stairs, it occupies an entire floor. One of the walls is mirrored—there's my shaved head—and the place resembles a dance studio. I have been ordered by Max to purchase a pair of cheap canvas slippers for the class and I slip them on to my feet. In sweatpants and a tee shirt, I am ready to get my Bruce Lee groove on.

Master Chu appears to be in his sixties. Wrapped in a dark blue ghi, he is small and wiry, with long graying hair that falls to his shoulders. His manner is autocratic and Max, normally garrulous and blustery, is deferential as he introduces us. The teacher seems distracted. There are fifteen other students there for the class, both men and women, and they are standing around talking, stretching, warming up. They are nimble, athletic, most around my age. It is not an unfamiliar environment to me. They remind me of dancers.

The college I attended had an excellent dance department and I took a class as an undergraduate. More recently, while in graduate school, I took some classes at Alvin Ailey Dance Studio—an excellent place for a heterosexual male to meet arty women—so when it comes to jumping around a room, I am not entirely without experience although, I hasten to add, I am basically without talent. But that is neither here nor there since today my physical aesthetic must please no one but me.

After a couple of warm-up exercises, Master Chu starts to teach the movements. Tai chi is considered a soft martial art, one applied with internal power. This distinguishes it from the hard martial arts, and their intended purpose of incapacitating an opponent. Tai chi evolved with the principles of Chinese wisdom traditions, particularly Taoism and its yin and yang duality. Since yin and yang is about balance, and I have managed to get completely out of balance, the practice appeals to me on a profound level. For this reason, it attracts people with little or no interest in martial arts, a group of which I am a member. When the karate movie phenomenon came and went, I barely noticed. I want the calm and the clarity, not the ability to break a cinder block with my forehead.

Individual routines are known as forms and they are comprised of a series of linked movements, what a dancer would call a combination. The movements are characterized by the use of leverage through the joints based on coordination in relaxation rather than tension. All of this allows the chi boundless free movement and the resulting happy, healthy life the free movement of chi provides.

The form Master Chu is attempting to teach takes about three minutes for him to demonstrate. Three minutes of continuous movement. Three minutes of continuous *graceful* movement. His arms and legs coordinate in a slow, hypnotic motion. Hands and feet continuously moving, he shifts his weight from one leg to the other, his body gyrating at a pace that is at once relentless and meditative. Master Chu is mesmerizing. There's no way I will be able to do this. But I am here to change my life and apparently you can't do that if you're not willing to flail around like a spastic dervish.

Master Chu finishes his demonstration and now it is our turn to ape his impossible to follow movements. He stares at us, hands on hips, his gaze a laser. Desperately trying to access my inner Baryshnikov, I place my feet shoulder-width apart, turn my legs out, dip one knee, lift an arm, start to pivot . . . and get completely lost. But Master Chu is patient and demonstrates again and again.

I always start at the beginning and each time, by focusing more intently and increasing my concentration, I am able to link the discrete movements together, get slightly further in the form, closer to some kind of ragged approximation of what Master Chu is attempting to impart.

And I completely forget that I'm sick.

It is difficult to recall whether the part where I move my right arm, elbow bent, palm up, is to the right or the left and is it linked with the part where I lift my right knee or the part where I pivot on my left hip? I concentrate mightily and after the first hour I manage a series of consecutive moves that, when strung together, take about forty seconds to perform. I am beginning to think I might actually be able to link three minutes of this. Already I feel my meridians opening.

I sign up for a series of ten classes.

Walking uptown after my first class, Max tells me about a more hard-core version of qigong called nei gong. Master Chu is teaching a nei gong workshop the following Saturday and he strongly suggests I sign up for it. The idea behind nei gong is to do the same thing as tai chi only faster. Faster? That would be risking injury. But Max informs me there is an added benefit. "They use nei gong in the training of Neijia where the object is the mobilization and coordination of your internal energies toward a target."

Toward a target? Cancer cells, perhaps?

I return to the dojo the following weekend for Master Chu's three-hour nei gong workshop. In the version he teaches, the practitioner holds specific poses for lengthy periods of time without moving. I was a Boy Scout for one year and one of the several lowlights of the experience was the Memorial Day Parade. We were forced to march for several hours in our uniforms, then stand at attention in the hot sun, not moving a muscle, as patriotic music blared. It was like being North

Korean for a day. I didn't mind the music, but the not moving a muscle part was unpleasant in the extreme. How would it be possible for me to perform nei gong?

The center of Master Chu's nei gong teaching, the signal pose, is a posture known as Embracing Horse. Embracing Horse is deceptively simple. Stand with your feet shoulder-width apart, weight on the outside of your feet. Bend your knees slightly, in a semi-sitting position. Arms are then placed in front of you as if you are leaning forward in a saddle and embracing, yes, a horse. Make sure your fingers are loosely held, palms facing toward you.

If you're in good shape, this is easy to do for about a minute. It is less easy at two minutes, and by the time three minutes rolls around most people are ready to have oxygen administered. I was warned my knees would begin to shake, my arms would quiver, my breathing would become labored. I was told that when I develop the stamina to continue past three minutes and make it up to fifteen or twenty, the most surprising thing happens—I'll begin to sweat. Without moving. I don't see how this is possible.

I assume the position canted forward and try to find a comfortable place for my hands, away from my body, palms facing inward. I am embracing the horse. Pleased with myself, I hold the pose and wait for the pain. It does not take long to arrive. In thirty seconds my legs are killing me. Master Chu does not care. "More sit!" he barks, placing his palm parallel to the ground and miming a downward push. More sit? Is he kidding? My thighs are throbbing; they're burning and I've been doing it for less than a minute. Nonetheless, I comply and squat to a level he finds acceptable. Nei gong, it occurs to me, as I try to think of things to pass the time, is the perfect exercise in which to engage since its endurance aspect fits in with the combat imagery I am continually calling forth in my struggle.

Despite throbbing pain in my legs, I am able to hold this posture for nearly five minutes. I did not sweat, but my confidence is buoyed by being able to do it at all.

I leave the dojo high from having learned the technique, armed with a new secret weapon. I do the forms at home, and then follow them with a nei gong practice. I work at it for an hour a day. Embracing Horse comes slowly. I hold the position for five minutes, then seven, nine, fifteen. My legs shake and rattle, I breathe as if I am running up the stairwell of an apartment building, great beads of perspiration rolling down my face and neck. My whole body is vibrating, meridians opening, pulsating with chi energy that feels as if it's on the verge of bursting through my skin. It's almost as if I am molting in some way, a trembling chrysalis, shifting, morphing and turning into something else, perhaps something healthier, something that will not die soon. I am now a shaved-headed, meditating, would-be vegetarian practitioner of qigong. A month ago, I was someone else. I feel as if I have dashed into a phone booth and emerged cloaked in an entirely new, supercharged identity. All while standing completely still. It is one of the most extraordinarily vivifying sensations I have ever experienced. Within a month, despite my weakened state, I am able to hold the Embracing Horse pose for forty-five minutes, during which I am almost entirely in the present moment because I'm so suffused with the energy being generated by the practice that I can't think about anything else for more than a fleeting instant, and the way that feels comes as a huge relief. To consider the past with neither longing nor regret, and not allow myself to be consumed by worry about what lies ahead becomes the next goal. As an animating philosophy, this is hard to beat. Whether it is achievable is another matter.

I begin my practice at 7:00 A.M., about an hour before my daughter awakens since her presence will not allow for anything requiring quiet. I do it to the accompaniment of Indian music, amusing in light of the ribbing I've given my brother for his Indian affinities. I squat and hold the pose until rivulets of sweat are pouring off. If Allegra wakes up early, Susan leaps into the breach and keeps her occupied until the arduous routine is completed.

Of course, I have absolutely no idea if any of this is actually doing any good. But no matter. Set the course. Believe. Go. What other choice is there?

Embrace the horse.

* * *

"Would you like to visit Paris?"

We are in our Manhattan kitchen on an early August evening. Susan has arrived home from work and I have just finished drinking a horrible-tasting health concoction. After three cycles of chemotherapy my enthusiasm is dimming. I'm not sure whether it's chemically-related lack of energy, or I'm just depressed. But that morning I got a phone call from my agent who asked if I wanted to write the screenplay for a film set in France. He did not have to inquire twice. Was there a research budget? There was.

"I do," Susan said.

A week later we are staying in an apartment on Rue Blomet in the 15th Arrondissement. The place belongs to a high school friend who works as a lawyer at a European firm and is conveniently in London on business. Allegra is home with a babysitter. Susan's belly has taken on the contour of a croissant. This is only an interlude, a break from the regularly scheduled programming, but our presence in this city is an extravagant declaration of life. A few months ago I was blindsided and pulverized. Now I am part of a venerable literary tradition, the American writer in Paris. I'll walk in the steps of John Dos

Passos, Gertrude Stein, James Baldwin. Who cares that I'm here to research a werewolf movie?

Because my immune system is wavering as a result of the treatment, I have developed a furious case of pinkeye which I treat with eyedrops and sunglasses. That I can barely open my eyes without feeling as if someone is driving long needles into them is not going to stop me from enjoying a stroll along the Seine on the studio's dime. We will pretend that this is just a trip to Paris and a sharpened sword is not hanging over our heads.

The "research" for the movie consists of visiting the Musee D'Orsay to see the Cezannes, descending into Les Egouts (the sewers), and sitting on a bench in the Luxembourg Gardens reading a Georges Simenon novel, along with a great deal of eating. The Cezannes are endless and inspiring, and Simenon never disappoints, but the sewers are a bust. The attraction features a subterranean museum, a slide show, and an open trench of filth whose length we traverse, holding our noses against the revolting smell.

"Remind me why we came here?" Susan says, breathing through her mouth.

"Research."

"Can we research some *moules-frites*?"

After lunch we find our way to Les Catacombs in Montparnasse and finally drop into the underworld—my were-wolf is going to spend a great deal of time beneath the streets. A maze of long dark tunnels, deep underground. Moisture on the stone walls and the ceiling, gravel under our feet. Then, the jewels: what seems like miles of hallways lined with neatly stacked femurs, fibulas, tibias, and skulls, arranged in a manner meant to be pleasing to the eye. The earthly remains of gone monks.

"Do you think the monks had any idea they'd be used as interior decoration?" Susan asks.

"It's a little macabre," I say.

"I wish I could have a glass of wine," she informs me.

It will not surprise you that we visit Pere Lachaise Cemetery. Despite the presence of such luminaries as Gide, Proust, and Balzac, the one that consistently attracts a crowd is Jim Morrison and at least twenty people mill in the area when we arrive. The grave is wedged between four others and consists of a simple headstone with the inscription *Jim Morrison 1943–1971* and beneath that the Greek words *Kata Ton, Daimona Eaytoy*, which translate *as true to his own spirit*, a theme to which I am trying to connect. Sand is scattered over the gravesite.

"It looks like a giant ashtray," Susan observes.

Perhaps because of this there is a forest of upright cigarette butts planted at the Lizard King's feet, assuming he has been buried facing the right direction. Also, several pots of geraniums, a candle, some roses, and a hefty security guard who is there to control overzealous Doors fans. There is such a party atmosphere, you almost expect to see someone grilling sausages on a hibachi. While I was never a huge Doors person, it was easy to relate to the ardor with which Morrison lived his brief life and standing there I recall my mother's tense reaction to the poster on my wall.

In the grave he is safe.

But Jim Morrison's spirit rages.

* * *

Susan and I are back in Dr. Speyer's office. The pinkeye that tormented me in Paris has resolved. It is late summer and I have absorbed all the cancer books, eliminated alcohol, discovered the joys of carrot and wheatgrass juice, learned how to meditate, ingested Chinese herbs, and practiced tai chi every day. Now we are going to find out how the chemotherapy has been working. Six months pregnant and pear-shaped, Susan watches as Dr. Speyer runs his fingers up and down my neck like he's playing a particularly challenging Scriabin piece on an oboe. Then he is rooting around beneath my arms and points south. I am so nervous I can barely breathe. What will he say? They're bigger, I'm sorry; we're tripling your dose? They're gone, you're done, see you later? Waiting. Waiting. Waiting.

"The palpable tumors are shrinking," he says.

*THEY'RE SHRINKING!*

I nearly melt with relief. I am a supernova, a star, exploding brilliantly in the night sky; I am God, on a good day, Vishnu, Shiva, Ganesh, Jesus, Buddha, Moses, and the guy who plays the organ at Yankee Stadium, all the positive energy in the universe flowing through me in a warm, healing wave. I'm not sure I have ever felt this good. Exculpating evidence has been unearthed, and I am being removed from death row, my last meal uneaten, and thrust back into life. Even Dr. Speyer, nothing if not phlegmatic, says my response to the treatment has been excellent.

"There's only one complication," he says.

Complication is not a word I want to hear right now. "And that is—?"

"Your white blood cells have been knocked out."

"Which means—?"

"You don't have any. So, don't get sick, all right?"

Sure, no problem. Why would I get sick if I have *NO WHITE BLOOD CELLS!*

Dr. Speyer informs me that I have to take injections of a love potion called Neupogen so I can raise my white count to a point where I can get more chemo because although the palpable tumors are significantly less palpable, there is still a riot of malignancy within.

Beth the Nurse instructs Susan and me on the art of the skin pop. Auto-injection is a nonstarter for me, given my aversion to needles, so Susan is appointed wielder-of-the-hypodermic. She will give the first injection in the office. We have been together for six years now but have never had a moment that feels quite so intimate, so naked. Susan has no scientific predilections, no fond memories of doing labs, or performing experiments. Nor does she have any experience with intravenous drug use. The only thing more nonsensical than her waving a hypodermic needle around would be if *I* were waving one around. It does not feel natural to her, this injecting of a husband with a vial of Neupogen. But, as always, she is game. And please don't forget: tired, stressful job, mother of a toddler, and the baby inside her growing larger each day.

The best place to inject the needle, Beth the Nurse informs us, is the fatty tissue of the stomach. A lifelong ectomorph, I don't have a lot of fatty tissue there, but I am instructed to pinch my skin and create an inviting target. I do this and wait for my wife to swoop in and stick me.

One of the greatest television shows of all time is *The Honeymooners*, a black-and-white 1950s sitcom starring Jackie Gleason and Art Carney that I discovered on late night television in my twenties. Gleason was Ralph Kramden, a Brooklyn bus driver, and Carney played Ed Norton, his sewer-worker pal. As a comedy team, they are among the best in history. One of my favorite bits involves them preparing to play golf for the first time. They are a couple of working stiffs and have no real idea of how this is done, but Ralph, as always, assumes he knows what to do and instructs Ed. Each man holds a club.

"Address the ball," Ralph says.

"Hello, ball," Ed says.

Art Carney then proceeds to prepare to hit the ball. He bends his knees, he flexes his arms, he swivels his neck. Then he does all of it again under his pal's increasingly impatient gaze. Still not satisfied, he begins to go through his routine one more time when Gleason, having lost all patience, bellows, "WILL YA HIT THE BALL, NORTON!?"

I picture Ed injecting Ralph in some long ago black-and-white doctor's office, *Ralph Gets Cancer: A Very Special*

*Episode.* I am grateful Very Special Episodes did not exist in the 1950s.

Susan is like Ed Norton with the syringe. She steps toward me, she steps back. She straightens her arm, she bends it. She giggles, she groans. Meanwhile, I am standing there worried the skin on my stomach will bruise because I am pinching it for so long. I want to yell, "Will ya hit the ball, Norton!"

After much ado, Susan finally introduces the needle to my flesh and manages to inject the drug. I barely feel it. The room is suffused with a profound sense of accomplishment. We feel as if we have just climbed K2.

I am becoming more and more confident of my ability to beat the cancer. My focus is strong and I feel good. I've made substantive changes in my daily habits and I am encouraged by the early results (and haunted by the words *it tends to recur*). Still, I am too easily prey to stress and irritability but very aware of their deleterious effects—that very awareness is draining—so I try to control my responses.

We are staying at Dad's house for a few days. This morning, I have to give myself an injection since Susan is out with Allegra.

I repeat: give *myself* an injection.

This would not have been possible a month earlier. But I do it without hesitation, grabbing the skin on my stomach, pinching, inserting the needle, and pressing down on the syringe. You would think I were a heroin addict so deft am I with the works.

Later, in front of my father's house, I settle into the Embracing Horse posture. As I start to perspire I notice the landscaping, the rolling lawn, towering old-growth trees, the rhododendrons standing like sentinels by the front door. My mother had a thing for rhododendrons. They were in front of each house our family lived in, the one on Brite Avenue, the one on Dolma Road, and now here. I can't see one without thinking of her. Now there are rhododendrons on either side of her headstone.

I spend most of the weekend curled up in my head. I burn with love for my wife and daughter. I also I burn when I urinate, only differently. My burning love is far preferable to my burning urethra. I am learning about side effects, two words that have always been an abstraction to me. I want to live with them for a long time—my wife and daughter, not the side effects. When the new baby arrives in November, I want to feel the pure joy in that and not the nagging undertow of my disease. If Dr. Strauss the Lymphoma King believes it can be cured, even if he is equivocal and lacks enthusiasm for this pronouncement, then so do I. Again, I resolve to do everything within my power to be around when the cure is discovered.

That night, Susan and I talk about moving out of New York City. Prior to our current circumstances, we had discussed California as a possibility. That seems too radical right now. The suburbs? That won't work either. And I don't know why I think moving is going to help. It's like changing the channel. One minute you're watching the detectives, the next it's doctors or lawyers. Wherever you are, you're still you.

But is that true? You are the same carbon-based life form you were in Prospect Park as you walk down a path on the island of Java. But perhaps the Javanese surroundings exert a pull that will have psychological ramifications. And perhaps those psychological ramifications will have somatic manifestations. All of which is a fancy way of saying perhaps you'll feel better.

# PART 4
## In Which We Light Out for the Territory

S usan was pushing Allegra's stroller down Amsterdam Avenue when a homeless person spat on her. *Spat.* On Susan. That this scabrous expectorator lived a rough, tragic existence there can be little doubt, and it was likely a series of bad breaks both in DNA and opportunity led him to launch a gob of spittle at a stranger. Ordinarily, that is the kind of thing she would have sloughed off.

But life is different now.

New York City has always exerted a gravitational pull. For the first few months after I graduated from college, I commuted from my parents' house to my copyboy job at the New York *Daily News* but by January had saved enough money and moved to an apartment on Bleecker Street in the West Village. Other than my early Los Angeles interlude, during which I pined for the city every hour of every day, I lived at various addresses in Manhattan for thirteen of the next fifteen years. I was a pure, lifelong New Yorker, never thought I could live anywhere else. I never thought I would *want* to live anywhere else. But things change. On an average day, the city is an ambient assault. The endless loop of noise from vehicles, construction sites, or the guy upstairs who wears cowboy boots twenty-four hours a day and is not familiar with the word *rug*, the aggressive jostling of the endless crowds, the piquant summer scents combining shades of rot from sources seen and sensed, taken together can tremble the ground on which a sturdy person stands. What a New Yorker thinks of as typical might send an Atlanta native into anaphylactic shock. But even the hardest of hard-core New Yorkers, the kind who remember the old Penn Station, who lived through the city-on-fire years, the kind that disdain summer getaways and can be seen reading the *Village Voice* in Tompkins Square Park on a sultry August day, the kind that have already decided to die in their rent-controlled apartments eating Chinese takeout directly from the container and watching public access cable, even members of that select group can't withstand everything. When your defenses, physical or otherwise, have been breached, the myriad charms of Manhattan can overwhelm. New York City is not a healing environment. As a place conducive to the regeneration of healthy cells, it does not rank high.

In sober tones we speculate. If Susan quits her job to move, we will be temporarily dependent on my screenwriting income and although this might imply a future of coupon clipping if not foraging in the forest, that is not the case. After the diagnosis, I stopped writing for an interval of self-pity and what psychologists call "existential distress." This went on for three days before exhausting itself in the manner of a storm. Realizing that I would not be struck dead that week, I collected myself and moved forward. Since then, I've been working on a pilot that I sold based on a play I wrote and just booked another screenwriting job. As long as I don't die, we'll be all right. Strangely, I don't feel resentment. It's happening; let's deal with it. Might this be magical thinking? Right now, that does not matter.

Having grown up in what Cheever imitators and writers of novel jacket copy refer to as "the leafy suburbs north of New York City," I had vowed to never return. I was not going to bring my children up in world of pasty Metro-North commuters.

That leaves the country.

I caught the tail end of the 1960s, which was characterized

by, among other things, a hippie-driven back to the land movement that made a fetish of simple rural living. There was a
rejection of the urban in the dominant culture that led large
groups of kids from towns like Great Neck to move to places
like Colorado. Western fashions were everywhere and all who
were around then recall the remarkable and deeply unfortunate popularity of the fringed buckskin jacket. Communes
sprouted like psilocybin mushrooms. Jug bands and jug wine
appeared. Someone named Country Joe was a rock star.
Canned Heat had a hit with a song called "Goin' Up the
Country."

I never bought into the back-to-the-country idea. Trees and
mountains are fine, but it's not as if I need to live among them.
I am the city. Asphalt runs through my currently overtaxed,
abused, and jaded veins.

But now the country beckons, hums, sings. It might be dull,
but it will be picturesque and have the added advantage of
being calm in the extreme. While the suburbs were boring too,
they are crammed with people who are oriented primarily
toward the city. This imbues them with an inchoate anxiety
manifesting in status obsession, child obsession, a fixation on
their lawns and flower beds, and gnawing confusion about
how they ended up in the suburbs. The country, fingers
crossed, will be anxiety-free. That should more than make up
for the unavailability of milk at 3:00 A.M. Moreover, it represents an action, not being passive, doing whatever is in our
power to move forward and create a sense of fleetness, of optimism. It's harder to hit a moving target.

But where to live?

Our first summer together, Susan and I rented a house in
Montauk. The memories of that time are happy ones so we
drive out there to look around. We see some lovely cottages
but it occurs to us that the Montauk of January has little in
common with the Montauk of July and we decide to keep

looking. We go to Connecticut to poke around. The towns in Litchfield County are closer to the city than Montauk but the place feels more precious than we remembered, an entire geographical area designed for a magazine layout. Finally, we settle on Cold Spring, New York.

Cold Spring is a picturesque town with a slightly tatterdemalion air, fifty miles north of New York City on the Hudson River. The schools are acceptable, if not ones that magnetically draw fleeing urbanites, and our daughter can enroll in the nearby Montessori program, situated in the quaint home of its owner, Miss Connie, a local fixture. No one within a New York City zip code would have the nerve to call herself *Miss Connie*, it being an entirely too Beatrix Potter a moniker. But we are about to no longer be New Yorkers, so the Montessori teacher having a name you would expect to be followed by . . . *and the Tale of the Industrious Bunny* is something we like.

The town itself, not much more than Main Street and a spur, is a stop on the Hudson train line which will allow us easy access should we find ourselves missing the urban pleasures, like sushi or medical care. There is a supermarket that doesn't quite live up to the billing, a video rental store, whose collection an East Village cineaste would laugh at (although Lou Gossett Jr.'s entire oeuvre is represented), a post office, and a suspicious number of antique shops. The local breakfast/lunch hangout is a place called Karen's Kitchen, run by Karen, warm and welcoming, a curly-haired ex-New Yorker. Cold Spring feels like a town far more than an hour away from the city. Other than the wide Hudson River booming past the bottom of Main Street, it could be Vermont.

We sign a one-year lease. I think of the old television show *Green Acres*—coincidentally, the name of the elementary school I attended—that starred Eddie Albert and Eva Gabor as New Yorkers who went rural.

A snippet of the theme song rings in my ears:

*You are my wife! Goodbye, city life!*

I'm still having treatment, and Susan is ever more pregnant. Now we're moving further away from the hospital, her doctor, my doctor. There's something a little crazy about this plan. It comes back to the idea of control. Moving to Cold Spring is a choice we can make of our own volition. Illness wags its finger—no, no, no—and denies one's agency. Leaving our old life behind reasserts it. It's an announcement to ourselves and the world that going forward things will be different. But yes, definitely a little intemperate.

The house we are renting is a white elephant on several acres along a dirt road. The backyard slopes into the woods that surround the property on all sides. We can't see our neighbors, something I love. The house is what would be called, were it for sale, a "fixer-upper"; in this case—like Dresden was a fixer-upper after WW II.

But that is not something we have to worry about. Upon signing the lease the ferret-faced landlord who is around our age and has a slippery quality assures us that all the appliances are in working order. He departs with a jaunty wave and we assure ourselves we are ready for life without a building superintendent. But an asthmatic washer/dryer, a dishwasher ready for last rites, and a stove that upon being examined by the gas company is summarily condemned let us know that we are not entirely correct in this assessment. In a dramatic touch, the gas company inspector wraps a piece of yellow hazard tape around the stove, as if it were a crime scene. Susan is now nine months pregnant, bursting, impatient, and this aggravation is most unwelcome. I reflexively pick up the phone to call the super, but the super in Cold Spring is like a phantom limb, something you sense is there but alas, is not. Ferret Face tells us not to worry, it will all be fixed. It turns out he is also a liar. But we don't know that yet. We're just thrilled to be living in the country, away from all that old stress, even as we cope with the spanking new stress being caused by our landlord who is beginning to rouse my sleepy inner Bolshevik.

On a positive note, we are visited regularly by a herd of inquisitive deer that periodically emerge from the woods, saunter insouciantly across our yard, and disappear back into the trees, transfixing Allegra, whose previous experience with wildlife has been confined to the squirrels and pigeons of Central Park. At bedtime, I conjure a story called *Allegra and the Talking Deer* in which she interacts with these enchanted creatures and deliver a command performance of a new version every evening at bedtime.

We explore the area, the hills and towns, the winding roads and the expansive vistas, many of which still resemble 19th century canvases painted by artists of the Hudson River School.

North of Cold Spring, nestled among the strip malls and fast food joints of Route 9, we discover a health food store. The place is too large for its inventory and the slightly under-stocked shelves suggest either a lack of commitment on the part of the proprietor or a lack of belief in the customer base. The supposedly fresh vegetables are fading fast. As for the owner, Ann, she does not look particularly well. Somewhere in her thirties and wearing a hemp pullover, she has the slightly spacey, patchouli-drenched, tie-dyed vibe of someone who has dropped too much acid and lost track of the decade. Her face is gaunt, her body emaciated. She barely fills out her clothes, which look like drapes suspended from a wire hanger. That her wraith-like appearance reminds me of my own is something I don't want to think about. But she's friendly and happily extols the virtues of macrobiotic living, of which she is an unconvincing advertisement. Still, I am intrigued.

On our first visit Ann introduces the concept of the skin brush. Skin-brushing, she informs me with the zeal of a terrorist, "removes the top layer of dead skin and circulates the blood." Fine, I think, eyeing the unimpressive tomatoes. Then she says, "Dry skin brushing is one of the most powerful ways to cleanse the lymphatic system."

"Really?" I say, suddenly riveted. The *lymphatic system?* Ann is playing my song.

"Oh, yes," she says, sensing a convert. "The lymphatic system carries waste material from the cells by the blood and the lymph. Did you know that?" I nod eagerly. We are now two lymph enthusiasts bonding. "So, you know that skin brushing stimulates the release of this material from the cells near the surface of the body, then they go to the colon and you poop them out."

I immediately purchase a skin brush.

I am so excited to have this new means of health maintenance I spring from the car when we get home. In the bathroom, I strip naked and begin buffing myself as if I were a vintage Corvette. Following Ann's instruction, I brush in long strokes from my outer extremities toward the center of my body. I raise an arm and brush from fingers to shoulder. I repeat the process with the other arm. Then the feet and legs. Then the back and head. I am tingling. In two minutes I have brushed every inch of my skin, said goodbye to millions of dead cells and communed with my lymphatic system in a way that announces how much it is cherished.

\* \* \*

My father calls to remind me that he still hasn't finished going through my mother's things and if I'm not too busy, perhaps I could give him a hand. His house is an hour away from our new home and I drive over the next day. Whether it's the move to the country, the chemically-induced multiplication of my white blood cells, or a growing sense of optimism now that the end of treatment is in sight, I can't say; but I'm feeling good.

Now we are sitting on the patio of his house, overlooking the lake, dotted with water lilies. Dad has done all the difficult work himself, giving away clothing items, donating the wig she wore after losing her hair, a short bob. Still, there are things he cannot bring himself to part with. A sheaf of papers is on the table in front of us and he is going through them. He holds something up, astonished. It is an old, tattered envelope. He removes a letter. I glance at it and see it is in his handwriting.

"I can't believe she saved this."

"What is it?"

A moment to collect himself, then: "I was flying out to California for a frozen foods convention. I don't even think Drew was born. The plane lost an engine and it looked like we might crash. It's the note I wrote your mother when we started losing altitude."

Handing me the page, he looks out over the lake. Birds twitter in the trees. A squirrel runs across the lawn. "Why didn't that plane go down? I got a gift of thirty-two years and I don't know where they went. I used to ask myself if I was put on this earth to sell blintzes." Milady's Blintzes was an agency account in his tyro days. "I wanted to be a writer."

"You did?"

"Come on, man. You knew that." I thought he had made a few half-hearted attempts. "I had rejection letters from every newspaper and magazine in the country."

"I had no idea."

"Sure, sure. Where do you think you get it from?"

"What happened?"

"You needed to eat. Don't feel guilty. I didn't have the talent."

My father's death would have come at the age I am now. *If* he had died. Instead he was given an additional decades-long reprieve. My Uncle Al was not so lucky. He died in 1960, in what was then the largest disaster in aviation history. Two passenger planes collided over Staten Island and everyone was killed. I wonder sometimes if Uncle Al's shocking fate contributed to my morbid streak. Although I experienced it at a remove, unlike my cousins, the idea that someone you love could be taken from you at any moment without warning was planted in me early. The ringing telephone, the relative's voice, the intimation of doom: just called to see how you were doing, they'll say. And I was worrying about death, I reflect, slightly breathless.

I don't know if I'll get that additional thirty-two years. I'd like to think I will, but who knows?

\* \* \*

In late October Susan's parents arrive for the birth. Her mother is chatty and her father hard of hearing. They have achieved perfect marital equilibrium. I refrain from asking if they are surprised I'm not dead.

Commuting back and forth into the city to work on a staged reading of my play *Red Memories* at Circle Rep, I leave Susan in the care of her parents. My sixth and final cycle of chemo is scheduled to begin the day after the last rehearsal for the play.

In Dr. Speyer's office, my heart is ready to take wing.

"You look great," he tells me. I beam like a kid who has just received a report card with straight As and await the rest of the good news. "So, we're going to give you two more cycles of chemo."

*Two more cycles?*

"Why?" Stunned.

I have been preparing myself for it to be over, goodbye to all that, and put the whole thing in the past.

"You're tolerating it so well," he says. "We thought we'd give you as much as you could take." I don't know whether to thank him or break a vase over his head. Ultimately, I am too grateful to argue. So I will take the poison, embrace the horse and the clean head, continue life as a patient, a soldier. Incongruously happy, I am the chemo poster boy.

Susan is late. The baby will not come. Unable to wait any longer, her father returns to Michigan. He is the town engineer in Paw Paw and needs to get back to work building bridges and roads. Susan's mother remains with us. We wait.

\* \* \*

Please welcome our son.

When Allegra was born, both of my parents were in the waiting room at the hospital. This time, my mother is gone and Dad is traveling in Cambodia.

Here is my journal entry for November 14, 1993:

*Gabriel Reid Greenland was born two days ago. 7 lbs. 13 oz. and all systems go. When his head popped out Dr. Moss, who was doing the delivery, asked if we thought it was a girl or a boy. We both said, "It's a girl." A couple of seconds later when Gabe, all purple and wrinkled, wriggled out the doctor said—this was before we could see anything—"You're wrong."*

*After Gabe was born I had to leave Susan's bedside so I could head down to NYU Medical Center for my fourth blast of chemo this week. I served my time on the needle then returned to Susan who just spent three hours in the recovery room next to a crackhead who was having her pregnancy terminated because her system could not tolerate it.*

*Sometimes I think I'd like to go away for a while but when I focus on the reality of that I know the one thing grounding me now is my family and I don't want to be apart from them at all.*

Soon after the birth our marriage is reduced to exchanges regarding laundry, food, cleaning, and, endlessly, child care. It's a loop familiar to all parents, one where you just hang on knowing it has to stop at some point. It feels as if we haven't had sex since the early days of the Ford Administration, other than a fumbling attempt that was abbreviated by Allegra pounding at the door like the secret police. While I recognize the current state of affairs is a result of the presence of small children, it is nonetheless frustrating. Allegra has been sleeping in our bed since she still does not like to be alone. She arrives and I depart. We pass silently, sleepily. I sleep in her bed so I can get more rest. My energy level is low because of the chemo and I require a good night's sleep. Susan requires a good night's sleep, too. The arrangement is suboptimal.

My mother-in-law has been with us for three weeks now. My organs (Liver? Kidneys?) feel sore, as if they have been absorbing body blows. Sick of the whole ordeal, I will have to grit my teeth just to get through the final two cycles.

Susan's sister Catie and brother-in-law George visit with their sons, Jake and Nick. For reasons I do not question and for which I am deeply grateful, these two boys, twelve and eight years old respectively, hold me in high esteem. Their presence is medicinal since I can actually do the things with them I can't do with my kids, a baby and a toddler. We spend a lot of time playing football, scoring touchdowns, dancing in the end zone. The nephews are a brilliant distraction and, since they are both inquisitive and generally of good cheer, superb company. I am sorry to see them leave.

Christmas comes and New Year's. We toast to a year that we fervently hope will be better.

But I am now consistently waking up in the middle of the night drenched in sweat, my tee shirt soaked. I have never had night sweats before. To wake up feeling like you've just run a 5K is unsettling. There are many reasons for this but here is the primary one: night sweats are a major lymphoma symptom.

Is the cancer really gone? Was the good report a mistake? I feel like every twinge is a tumor returned. When I look at the obituaries in the paper now, I read the second paragraph first.

This is where they often report the cause of death. "After a lengthy illness"—that can't *always* be cancer but it always feels like cancer to me. Brain tumor. AIDS-related something. Heart attacks, strokes, accidents. But why obsess? My son is developing a healthy pair of lungs and a joyful nature. Allegra is thriving. There are so many things going right, so much to be grateful for.

I see Dr. Speyer at his office. Susan is taking Gabe for his checkup so I am there alone, something I never like to do. Visiting your oncologist alone is like going into a haunted house by yourself. There are premonitions of death everywhere and something might leap out (bad test results) and scare you senseless. I am not brave enough to face this alone, but here I am. He feels around my neck for what seems like half an hour, thinking he has found a node. Ultimately, he determines it is the end of a muscle but panic crashes like thunder over my head as I imagine the medicine has stopped working. I look forward to completing the treatment with a mixture of happiness and dread. For all of my meditative practices and attempts to subtly shift my consciousness I am in deep fear of a recurrence right now.

*It tends to recur.*

I realize this is living in the future instead of occupying the present moment and so is antithetical to my new philosophy but there it is; the fear keeps peeking through the elaborate, well-designed, and—until recently, I believed—impermeable shield I've constructed. After my experience with Dr. Speyer I think about staying in town to see a movie or go to a museum before taking a qigong class but I am so unnerved that I go directly home.

I've upped my vitamin intake and added yeast tablets. We bought an industrial-strength juicer and carrot and apple juice, both heavy with antioxidants, are being consumed along with the juice of a raw potato at the rate of two quarts a day. My anxiety level appears to have spiked if that's possible, amazing given its already Himalayan heights. I'm not sure if it's because I'll be done with the treatment and will have nothing further to do as of next month or it's just the free-floating variety that periodically alights and is compounded by the current uncertainty. New permutations arrive daily. I am so consumed by unease about my health, work-related worry, a reliable staple, has vanished. There's a twinge in my lower right intestine—what the HELL is that?

\* \* \*

I get my left ear pierced and spring for a diamond earring. The diamond is meant to represent the clarity with which I now see things. It feels like a sturdy if slightly strained and self-conscious piece of symbolism. Still, I'm committing to it.

It is the dead of winter, the days when April seems a year away. I am in the last week of chemo now—*THE LAST WEEK!*—and feel completely shot, a burned-out engine. Four days down, one to go. A final round and it's over, I hope for good. A man sprayed a Long Island Rail Road car with gunfire earlier in the week, killing five people. Life seems increasingly arbitrary. The shooter was an African-American who said he didn't like Caucasians or Asians. This is alarmingly close to I don't like Mondays. The Dadaist artist Tristan Tzara created poetic juxtapositions by pulling words randomly out of a hat, as good an explanation as any for how the universe works.

The January winds bluster outside my Cold Spring window as I recline in a steaming bathtub reading a magazine. Nat King Cole's voice drifts up from the kitchen. Bliss, pure and steaming.

At lunch with my friend Rick on the Upper West Side, he asks me to define happiness, after he covers his intellectual base by characterizing it as a dumb question. What makes me happy is seeing Allegra toddle into the kitchen in furry slippers.

Making Susan laugh. Hearing the Velvet Underground play "All Tomorrow's Parties." What makes me happy now is that I have learned to consistently appreciate the small change, the pennies, nickels, and dimes that comprise our days.

Rick is thinking about getting married but he's worried that marriage is the death of hope. I tell him that it's not the death of hope at all. It's the death of the romantic illusion that life is an endless peak experience. Rick asks about the diamond earring. I trot out the line about how the diamond represents the clarity with which I now see things and notice that the words feel a little ridiculous. To his credit, Rick does not laugh. Has cancer made me insufferable?

\* \* \*

After finishing my eighth cycle of chemotherapy, I exit the hospital and tap dance up First Avenue, vault over taxicabs, do somersaults off building walls. In my head. I am a chorus line of high-kicking Rockettes, an ecstatic solo. With luck this treatment will really, truly, *finally* be my last. So long needles, nausea, constipation, and other deflating side effects that would have brought a twinkle to the Marquis de Sade's eye. In two weeks I have a CAT scan. If that's clean I have a bone marrow scan. If *that* is clean I have reached the end of the process.

Dr. Speyer tells me the hardest part of going off chemotherapy is not being able to do anything for one's self. This does not sit well with me. Between a radical diet shift, vitamins, and qigong I feel like I have enough to keep me occupied on that front.

The woods outside my window are white. It's mid-afternoon but the metal gray sky gives the day a brooding cast. Snow lightly drifts down on our dirt road, on our village, on the Hudson flowing southward to the city of our former life. The day is ending. Darkness comes yet I am not frightened. Possibility rears its head. I don't want to feel elation yet, elation is a bridge too far. If more cycles of chemo are required I'll lace up the gloves and climb back in the ring.

I have ceased reading newspapers. Why worry about things you can't do anything about? If the idea is to lower stress, then following world events is not going to help. I suspect this feeling will pass but right now I luxuriate in my ignorance. The lack of information flowing in jibes well with pastoral living. When the kids aren't screaming the quiet is almost voluptuous.

My nose is turning orange. This is because of all the beta carotene in the gallons of carrot juice I have ingested. It does not matter that there is no dignity in an orange nose.

* * *

Although my readership of print media was on hiatus during that time in Cold Spring, books remained a lodestone. In fleeting moments when both kids slept, I inhaled a contemporary novel about a group of students at an elite college who murder a peer. The story was diverting and well-told but I required stronger whiskey. For years I had resisted the narrative blandishments of the Kennedy assassination but I picked up *Libra* by Don DeLillo and this sent me swirling down the conspiratorial vortex where I inhaled half a dozen books on the subject. Why did this material suddenly appeal? Perhaps it was because the last few months of my life were about the wanton destruction of reliable patterns and assassination buffs are forever trying to establish them. Was I attempting to map a personal existence of which I could make sense by determining whether Kennedy was killed by anti-Castro Cubans, the Mob, or a lone gunman? It seems like the most logical explanation. Conspiracy theories are like religion. Those who obsess over them seek to superimpose the geometry of understanding over what often appears to be chaos and so develop a world-view to which they can hold fast.

And like religion, conspiracy theories offer the comfort of an assumed logic. However terrifying or incomprehensible something might appear, at least there is an explanation. For a while, I had a complex theory about what happened in Dealey Plaza but now I can't remember what it was.

When my assassination fever broke, I dove into *The Death of Ivan Ilyich*. Safe in the knowledge that my own death was not imminent, I was enthralled by Tolstoy's brief novel in which he limns the moment-to-moment consciousness of a dying man. I charged through the text as if it were a mystery which, in a sense, it is. Will the titular character expire in a state of ignorance about his predicament or glean a sliver of understanding? The average life expectancy when Tolstoy published the novel was forty-one years, so while this was not exactly a case of *Ivan, c'est moi*, it was not far off. Rubbernecking poor Ivan Ilyich's demise, I congratulated myself on having so recently dodged the scythe and Tolstoy's book provided a front row seat to what I had missed. The appeal of this particular work might seem counterintuitive given what I had just been through. Perhaps it would have been more comforting to read about basketball or the life of Duke Ellington, but the gossamer thread that tethers me to this world had been frayed and I wanted to embrace the opportunity to better comprehend what was going to be, in the end, unavoidable. Ivan Ilyich does not understand death. It happens to him. To not replicate his experience was now a goal.

Of humankind, Samuel Beckett cheerily wrote: "They give birth astride of a grave."

We are already living through our own death. Even you, Reader.

\* \* \*

In old weepies like the classic *Mildred Pierce*, based on the novel by James M. Cain, a character who is fated to die of an illness will cough. They might not expire in that reel, but death is not far off. Mildred is a hard-working woman who battles a man's world to provide material advantages for her children. She deserves some luck, but life has other ideas. Mildred's younger daughter coughs, and soon the girl is in movie heaven. The clinical designation of this phenomenon is "movie cough" and its raspy sound invariably portends a dire turn of events. Having only just finished treatment, dire events are still in the forefront of my mind.

On a winter morning I am in Gabe's room changing his diaper when he coughs. He's been coughing for the last few days and it is starting to seem like it may be more than just a cough. I don't like the sound of it at all. With him lying naked on the changing table, I think of God summoning Abraham to the top of Mount Moriah where he will have the opportunity to prove his faith by sacrificing Isaac, and Abraham's willingness to kill his son. If God asked me to prove my faith by harming this perfect and vulnerable boy, I would tell God with all due respect to go fuck Himself. I'm pretty close to doing that anyway even though I don't believe in Him. Then I think of my father, who years earlier saw me naked and vulnerable, and can only imagine what has lately been going through his mind as he has witnessed my struggle and been unable to protect me.

We haven't been in Cold Spring long enough to have a pediatrician we trust so Susan and I decide to drive into the city to take Gabe to the doctor. We get Allegra dressed to travel and wrap Gabe up. The weather has warmed slightly which means the snow has changed to cold rain. I'm feeling ill on the drive into town, hot, sweaty, and a little light-headed. I grip the wheel and stare straight ahead, willing us to our destination. At the pediatrician's office we wait to be granted an audience. When the pediatrician finally examines Gabe he does not like what he sees and sends us to the hospital. Apparently, his cough is not just a cough but a serious respiratory ailment. We look at each other. What next? I feel faint but keep pushing onward. My son is sick. I can't be sick, too. I've already been sick. I can't possibly be sick again. What kind of father does that make me?

Gabe gets checked into the NYU Medical Center where I am beginning to feel as if I should buy a condo. The doctor examining him takes a look at me, says, "You don't look so great either," and "suggests" I see my doctor immediately. This is not something you want to hear when visiting your son's pediatrician. Dr. Speyer is not there that day, so I am seen by another physician thereby ending my streak of not seeing a doctor at nearly ten days. I don't mind, though, since at this point I sense something unexpected and potentially dire is happening. The doctor on call takes my temperature. It is 102—anything above normal can be dangerous now—so he immediately checks me into the hospital. I have stopped the injections meant to raise the white blood cell count and my immune system is incapable of fighting off an infection.

Any infection.

As a rule, the patient does not want to leave home without an immune system.

It does not escape me that bad outcomes can arise from the treatment rather than the disease. In obituaries, a genre in which I could now teach a college course, a word often seen is *complications*. Complications of pneumonia, of AIDS, of cancer. I now had complications.

Another doctor, one named Anton Chekhov, who between seeing patients did a little writing, famously stated that if you show a gun in the first act, it had better go off in the third act. Having no white blood cells is a Chekhovian gun. I had not realized that when our latest adventure began.

The medical professionals put me in co-op care where a friend or relative stays and pitches in since the doctors think you won't need a lot of attention. Drew is slated to be my roommate since Susan is performing a similar function for our baby who is in another wing of the same hospital.

Drew arrives and helps me get settled in the room, a relatively easy task since I didn't expect to be there and so have nothing with me. He is good-humored and calm, and very welcome. I am deeply grateful for his presence. Years of meditation have subtly altered his DNA. Calmness and serenity radiate from him. We sit silently in the room for a few minutes after he arrives. I sip water, trying to hydrate. My mind drifts to the summer I graduated from college. Drew has just finished his freshman year and the two of us are camping together in Glacier National Park in Montana. Glacier Park is a grizzly bear habitat and being deep in the backcountry we're hyper-conscious of this. A clear July morning, ten miles from the nearest road on a wilderness trail outside of Red Eagle Lake headed for Medicine Grizzly Lake. We're singing, clapping, and yelling "Yo" a lot (remember, this was the '70s). The premise is don't startle the bears—a surprised bear is an agitated bear hence the stomps and hollers. Not only are we creating this cacophony with our hands, feet, and lungs but we've also attached bells to our hiking boots. And the bells are *RINGING* for the saints. Any bear within five miles is going to know we're in the neighborhood. A deaf bear is going to hear us. We see a lot of fresh bear tracks and some bear scat but no bears. We proceed deeper into the wilderness. The hike goes along at a crisp pace for the first six miles. We stop by a stream and wolf some trail mix and water, then head up Triple Divide Pass, beyond which, in a basin-like valley, lies our destination. The ascent begins gradually, winding through fields and meadows, past an explosion of wildflowers, purple, blue, yellow, red, and into the thick underbrush. It's warm and the sun shines on us, keeping our bodies warm—a necessity for mountain climbing.

Triple Divide Pass is comprised of three peaks, all over

seven thousand feet. Its name is actually a misnomer since you don't actually pass through it but go up and over it. And by up, I mean way, way up, where the elevation is roughly ten thousand feet and the thin air is frigid at night. This route comes as something of a surprise since we had anticipated going around gradually as opposed to up quickly. We dig in, legs pumping, and begin to climb. About a mile from the top I find myself short of breath. My heart begins to tom-tom, knocking against my chest. At twenty-two years old, you are generally not conscious of even having a heart, so this is an alarming development. At first, I'm resting every few minutes, panting like a sheepdog in August, waiting for my energy to regenerate. But as we climb higher and higher and my body is increasingly fatigued the rests come more and more frequently until I can't walk ten feet without stopping where I place my hands on my knees and suck air. Every step takes superhuman effort. My entire body feels wasted. The peak, despite my best efforts, appears to be receding. I feel monumentally frustrated and, worse, sick. Every movement seems to double my heart rate and breath intake. Now when I rest between my brief exertions, I collapse to the ground.

Drew is in fine shape, having done a wilderness course earlier in the summer and his patience is remarkable. On stone legs, I push forward. After what seems like hours we reach a point about a hundred yards from the top. My pack has just broken and happy for an excuse to take another break, I sit down to mend it, gasping for oxygen. While my fingers work the strap, I start to feel woozy, as if I'd just smoked a joint. Looking around, I see an icy blue glacial lake about half a mile below us. We're above the timberline, nearly in the clouds. A mountain goat casually regards us from a short distance away as he pokes his head through the smaller rocks looking for sustenance.

The sun grinds hot on my neck and I start to shiver. The

temperature could not have been much less than sixty-five degrees and I am shaking, rattling in my hiking boots. Drew stands in front of me with his pack on to create a shadow in which I can sit. He takes out a wool shirt and a down vest and puts them on me. Still, I shiver. We haven't eaten lunch and are burning energy like a rocket. My body has begun to consume its own heat. I am experiencing exposure, the first stage of hypothermia, a potentially fatal development. Drew sits down directly next to me to transfer his body heat. After a few minutes of this we decide to try and get me to the top. I attempt to eat a bite of cheese for energy and nearly spit it up. The idea of food is nauseating. Leaving my pack on the ground, I grab my brother's arm and stagger behind him to the summit struggling for breath as if someone had strapped a keg of beer to my chest. By the time we make it to the grassy knoll on the pinnacle, I feel like I am slipping into unconsciousness. Drew lets go of me and I fall to the ground. I am so weak I can barely curl up to keep warm. He stays with me for a few minutes then hikes back to retrieve the packs. Since I have become luggage, they were more than he could carry. I feel like Dustin Hoffman in *Midnight Cowboy* during the scene where he tells Jon Voight he can't walk anymore. When Drew returns I am crying, out of shame, out of gratitude. Never before have I felt like such a complete waste of bones and flesh. Sitting on top of Triple Divide Pass, one of the grandest vistas in North America spread out before me, I have finally reached the top and instead of leaping, fists in the air, roaring triumphantly to the clouds below, I am crumpled in a pathetic heap. And here is Drew saving my life and that makes me blubber more. Drew wraps his sleeping bag around me and eventually I stop shivering. We stay up there for an hour and when strength slowly returns to my limbs head down the other side of the pass, me with the sleeping bag draped over my shoulders like a blanket and Drew humping both of our backpacks. Pretty soon I am strong enough to "yo" around the curves in the trail and we finally make it to the campsite at the lake.

It is said that this kind of experience builds character but that is not true. This kind of experience reveals it. Drew acted with more calm, poise, and aplomb, more character, than I had ever seen a human being exhibit in real life. It snowed heavily on the peak that night. If there hadn't been anyone there to drag me up and over and warm me up I surely would have died.

I am seated in a wheelchair and Drew is ready to resume his role as my savior seventeen years after last being called. Again, I am ready to keel over. Again, death lurks. Again, my brother is here. I'm not sure what I've done to deserve a wife and a sibling like the ones I've been given.

The room is shadowed, the lamps weak. Several stories above the street, it feels like we're underground. It is nearly time to get an IV antibiotic. I rise to go to the bathroom, a task I convince myself I can do without assistance. As I emerge and make for my wheelchair, I am overcome with dizziness and nausea. I suddenly notice I am drenched in sweat. I sit down because it seems I am unable to walk. Again, my legs are stone. Again, we are short of the summit. Again, I am fading into nothingness. Drew wheels me to the elevator and we ride one floor up where the doctor on call takes my temperature: 105. My white blood count is around 100, roughly 1/40th normal. Physically, I am obliterated. Life is seeping out of me.

Then the doctor, in his forties with dark, curly hair looks at me with an ominous expression and utters the following words: "I don't want to alarm you, but you're in an unstable condition."

An *unstable condition.*

He has utterly failed in not alarming me but I am too sick with terror to berate him for his poor word choice. So, not only am I in an unstable condition, but I am there without an immune system. It is starkly clear that the fever could get out of control. At least he left out the implicit *and you could die.* I have been riding this bus long enough to figure that out for myself. The dizziness again, this time longer lasting, sickening. A chasm opens and I am slipping into it. This could be my last night on Earth. Is this how it's going to end, in a hospital with a fever? Quietly, drifting, warm, hot, black, nothing. I am conscious enough to be scared but I won't go to pieces.

Breathe. Breathe. Breathe.

You're not going to die, you can't die; it would be ridiculous. But life can be ridiculous. At times that is all that it is. A child is born with fetal alcohol syndrome. A healthy young woman perishes in a car accident. Shit, as they say, happens.

The doctor immediately places me in the Intensive Care Unit where, petrified, I lie in bed willing the medication to kick in. I have faith in these doctors, in what western medicine can often do. I am here because of western medicine; that is what has made the tumors vanish. I try to relax and not watch the IV drip, drip, dripping. My thoughts careen from Susan to Gabe. How could we both be in the hospital at the same time? I am overcome with guilt that I can't help Susan now, but the guilt is washed away by panic—all this while having a fragile hold on consciousness, which flickers in a wash of fear, and intense longing.

I think of Ivan Ilyich. Am I ready?

The effects of the swoon dissipate and a few hours later I am starting to feel what passes for normal, which is to say weak and feverish, but not blacking out. My limbs are useless, the strength to leave the bed absent. Broken, I lie in the ICU for two days on constant IV antibiotics and hydration drips. Eavesdropping on the other patients; listening to the radio. Susan arranges for Allegra to stay with friends so she can remain with me. She periodically finds her way to another part of the hospital where Gabe is being treated. The stress on

Susan is difficult to imagine as she pinballs between the two of us. Catie flies in from Michigan to help look after Gabe. My sister-in-law's arrival shores up the foundation and helps to keep everything from further deteriorating. Her kindness is a gift.

Leonard comes to visit.

"Babe," he says.

"Babe," I whisper.

His presence temporarily lifts my spirits although I am still too weak to walk across the room. I barely have the strength to talk so he tells me news of his latest gig, hosting a radio show where he interviews comedians. This one is hilarious, that one a wonderful guy. I can barely smile but I am so pleased he is there, so grateful for our friendship.

A little improvement, and then more, until finally I can get out of bed and walking to the door and back doesn't feel like crossing the Sahara. The hospital is home to Gabe and me for a week although we do not see each other even once.

I am sitting in the day room with a magazine. The ability to concentrate has not returned so I spend most of the time watching the other patients. Weak, dried up, we are an uninspiring group, teetering on the precipice. One woman, small, birdlike, barely eighty pounds, bent but somehow ambulatory, looks like she's been dead for three days and no one has had the heart to inform her. But these are my people. I am one with them, near ghosts, afraid to glance in the mirror.

Susan comes to see me whenever she is not with Gabe. On the sixth day, we are seated in the day room. I notice the weather has improved considerably. I ask her how our son is doing.

"He's all right now, but it was touch and go."

"Touch and go?" My voice cracks. I have not heard this before. "What do you mean?"

"That lung infection turned out to be RSV—"

"Which is—?"

"Respiratory Syncytial Virus. Don't ask me to spell it."

"And—"

"The doctor says he's fine now," she assures me. "He's going home tomorrow."

I have no idea what to say to this other than I don't know how Susan has made it through the week. I get discharged from the hospital after having a second bone marrow aspiration, the results of which will be known in a week.

The four of us go home.

It feels like a Beatles reunion.

My strength slowly returns and I consider my appointment with Dr. Speyer next week. This is when he will tell me whether I am in remission, something he has not said yet.

He said, "You're improving."

He said, "The palpable tumors are shrinking."

What he has not said are the words I so desperately wanted to hear (Actually, those words are "You're cured" but I'm willing to settle right now). I feel as if I was about to cross the finish line of a marathon when a truck ran me over.

The woods around our house are thick with snow. I don't remember a winter like this since I was a child. Susan is sick now. Since the crises have momentarily subsided, she has the luxury of being able to break down. A fever and raspy coughing. But Gabe and I survived and this is not a movie cough. Susan will get well and unlike the characters in *Mildred Pierce*, we allow ourselves to believe in the possibility of a happy outcome.

* * *

In late January, there is a message on the phone machine, exactly the same way we learned of the diagnosis, informing us the bone marrow is clean—*Clean!* Healthy! Bursting with cells behaving as they're meant to behave, not racing fast cars down teeming streets, mounting sidewalks, mowing down innocent people. Cells that are happy to let you go about your life without worrying that they are engaged in violent insurrection—and no more treatment is needed. No more treatment? Weak in the knees, I could swoon.

Remission, at last. Stunned by good luck. Susan and I embrace. Acute bliss washes over me and I am momentarily without words. It's as if I'm being bathed in radiant light. It is a better feeling than any other because it portends the opportunity for more feelings. More life. We have fought this brutish monster side by side and at least for now—

Gaining control of myself, I start to call people since this is the kind of news you want to see in skywriting, white puffy letters one hundred feet high. My father's relief is unmistakable ("Oh, man, that is great, great news") and if Drew's ("Congratulations") is less overt if no less sincere—no one is moved to poetic heights—that hardly matters; it's easy to hear how pleased they are, how thrilled. Susan's family, our friends are all on the receiving end of calls that find me trying not to squeeze through the phone and pinch everyone's cheeks. I'm here, I survived, I want to scream, shout, bellow and hear the echo from canyon walls, the sides of buildings, from the moon, as I try to play it cool, hey, I knew it all along, didn't you, and fail miserably.

When the initial euphoria recedes, the reality of remission is not easily internalized. I feel as if a pardon has been granted by a mad monarch that might be revoked in a capricious moment. The out-of-the-blue nature of this onslaught caused a massive shift in perception: change can occur in a second. One moment you're healthy, the next someone says you have Stage 4 cancer and they're going to France.

*My Dinner With Andre* is a movie that largely, to this film critic, consists of two old friends gassing about what it means to be enlightened. The romantic one claims true enlightenment requires extreme experiences that tax the nervous system and challenge every precept. The more practical one posits that you don't have to trek to a mountain peak or partake of a tribal fertility rite or do anything out of the ordinary to achieve enlightenment. It could come, he maintains, by going no further than the corner of your street. For now, I have learned to take the second view. So much of our lives are comprised of things like brushing our teeth, raising a window shade, eating a strawberry, buying stamps, walking in the sun. When you realize that it is not just the extraordinary things we do that have a limit but that our ordinary moments are finite, too, those quotidian hours become suffused with a richness they may have previously lacked. Actually, that isn't accurate. Those fragments of time never lacked for richness. What was lacking was my ability to perceive it. Walking the dog can be a universe. This realization is a gift. Indeed, it can be exhausting; you can find yourself overwhelmed by acuity of perception and unable to cope, like Virginia Woolf who responded to this predicament by filling her pockets with rocks and walking into a river. But to perceive the sublime in the ordinary, the poetry in the mundane is to experience life as it must be inhabited if we want to say we have lived rather than simply existed. Do you disagree? Are you a mollusk? Of course not. I don't mean to imply that making a tuna sandwich is necessarily a celestial symphony, but a little more awareness never killed anyone, and please don't say:

Yes, but what about Virginia Woolf?

* * *

The exit interview with Dr. Speyer feels like graduation. He is cheerful, but noncommittal. Remember, he's not selling a cure, but remission. It's like being returned from the prison of illness to the civilian population but as a second-class citizen, one with a shadow no amount of sunlight will dispel. There must be something I can do, I say. The idea of being cast back into an existential void absent means that will allow me to define the struggle is almost too much to bear. Have I become strangely attached to my chemotherapy? Is that even possible? I experience a cognitively dissonant feeling not unlike that of a soldier who misses war because, however dangerous, chaotic, and deadly it may be, it was the boundary that had come to define his existence; and when that boundary dissolves everything begins to drift. Relief mixes with a wholly unforeseen incipient fear.

There's really nothing I can do? Dr. Speyer shrugs and tells me to come in for regular checkups. When I leave the doctor's office with his cheery cry of "Good luck!" ringing in my ears, I think: What now? My doctor who has cured me with his magical toxic potion believes I can't do anything at this point other than wait and see but he has so spooked me about the possibility of a recurrence that doing nothing, something for which I have no talent anyway, is not an option. I can perform qigong, eat a macrobiotic diet, brush my skin, and recite my dialectical version of prayer, but all that strikes me as not quite enough, half measures, a start, a beginning, but a path too strewn with unicorns and rainbows. All these things taken together lack the tincture of relentless assault I require. This is the quandary to end all quandaries. Do I just go about life with my tenuous sense of enlightenment and wait? There is a Hemingway short story called "The Killers" in which a man on the run takes up residence in a boarding house and waits for the hitmen who are coming to kill him. They made a movie out of it in which Sterling Hayden played the victim. He knows they're coming and has time to get away but he does nothing. Nothing! He just lies there on the bed. He poses, he pouts, and he waits. Will I be like Sterling Hayden, only less good-looking? Wait for the footfall, the knock, the bullets?

*It tends to recur.*
No one ever confused me with a Hemingway character.

\* \* \*

Absent Susan, it's hard to know how the story would have turned out. In the writers' room scenario I described earlier, the bad version was one where the main character gets cancer. An equally bad version is the one where the character's husband gets cancer while she is pregnant and already caring for a toddler. That would be, as the French say, *de trop*. There's another writers' room expression: "putting a hat on a hat." Susan's situation was definitely putting a hat on a hat. Despite the manifold burdens foisted upon her by the maniacal author of our untidy narrative, you have observed not only the grace with which she bore them, but the way she turned out to be an actual lifesaver. Before she could step into that role, however, she had to look after herself. And the way she looked after herself was not only good for her but good for me and, as an added benefit, deeply enriched the life of our family. Allow me to pitch that movie:

Act One:
A girl from rural Michigan, college theater major, moves to New York City after graduation, interns in the opera department at Juilliard, gets a job at a film studio, then as an assistant to a famous director. In her mid-twenties she enrolls in law school, passes the New York State bar on the first try, and gets hired as an associate at a "white shoe" law firm. In tailored power suits and heels, she works for Fortune 500 clients. She buys a metallic blue sports car and drives it to corporate headquarters where she puts in long hours. Marries a screenwriter and they have a baby girl. A desire to return to her showbusiness roots lands her in the legal department of a broadcast

network. In that capacity, she flies around the country leading sexual harassment seminars, attending depositions, appearing in courtrooms. In an era of big hair and bigger shoulder pads, she cuts a sleek, understated figure. She likes her colleagues, the money is good, the horizon bright. It's all very glamorous. And she's going to have another baby. Then her husband gets cancer and it comes with a sticky prognosis. She resigns from her job to care for him. The power suits are folded and packed, the high heels stowed. The expense account is a memory. They move to the country where it will be easier to live a healthy life.

Act Two:

A falling-down house in a Hudson River town. The formal dining room has been turned into an office. A shingle is hung—not actually but picture a shingle—and she's going to be a country lawyer. Office supplies are purchased. Stationery printed with her letterhead. A few weeks pass with no work but the hours are occupied with family obligations; organic juices need to be made every day, a toddler needs to be cared for, and she is now very pregnant. Her husband commutes to the city for chemotherapy treatments. A nanny is hired who quickly violates her trust by stealing a piece of the stationery and forging her signature on it to transact a bit of personal business. This adds to the already high level of stress. There is a confrontation, and she scolds the nanny. The nanny pushes back, shouts: You want blood? She does not want blood. Things are already too bloody.

She feels helpless, tired, scared.

One day, there is a ray of light: the first client, a woman in her sixties who wants a will written. She tries to oblige, consults legal manuals, scratches some notes. But life intrudes, children, husband. Calls from the client go unreturned. It turns out that the high-octane lawyer so recently jetting around the country, sleeping on high thread count sheets, and striking fear into the hearts of sexual harassers from Charlottesville to Sacramento has no idea how to write a will. The woman fires her. She takes it hard, yet paradoxically is somewhat relieved. She did not put herself through law school and then burnish her resume to wind up wasting away in some podunk town practicing parking ticket law. The hours pass. Days and weeks go by. New clients fail to materialize. Despair peeks in the window and observes her seated at the desk in the converted formal dining room, her belly now huge with the new baby, blonde head in hands. She longs to flee, but there is nowhere to go. She can't abandon her husband, their toddler, this life.

As a child, she had found solace in prayer so she volunteers at the food bank of a local Presbyterian church, attends Sunday morning services. But this does not address the underlying sense of things spinning out of control. She yearns for a private, numinous space to which she can retreat and commune with a larger universe, one without unceasing obligations, distractions, terrors. Even though her first encounter with meditation back in the city did not end well, the idea still appeals.

And so she lies on her back and begins listening to recordings of guided practices led by founders of the Insight Meditation Society. When she feels strong enough to sit upright, a zafu is purchased. She settles on to it, crossing her legs. She closes her eyes, relaxes, focuses on breathing. This time, when she becomes anxious or uncomfortable, she is able to stop and start as she likes, get off the cushion and get back on. Get off again, go make a cup of tea. Get back on.

I'm going to meditate, she says, and disappears to another part of the house. To her husband's amazement, she begins to do this regularly. Everyone knows someone who decides to study the clarinet, take up jogging, learn to knit, and does it with a passion until other things begin to interfere—cocktail hour, a diverting television show, napping—and life returns to what it was before their new enthusiasm took hold. This does not happen.

She gets ready for bed and her husband asks how long she meditated that day.

An hour, she casually reports. Like it's nothing.

Act Three:

Because her husband is writing movies for several west coast studios, the family moves to California where she passes the California bar exam and gets another high-paying legal job. The baby in her belly is now a toddler. She studies privately with a meditation teacher in Culver City, and then with his teacher in Pasadena, driving an hour in traffic each way for the privilege. East of Los Angeles, at a zendo in the San Gabriel Mountains, she attends her first silent retreat. It lasts for five days. On the zafu, the extended silence might not always be exquisite but it is often illuminating. She goes on more retreats, each one lasting a week or two. Once or twice a year she leaves home to meditate in this concentrated way. It allows her to slow down and focus; gives her the capacity to sit with strong emotions that used to overwhelm. It rejuvenates her. She invites women over to meditate in a group setting. Living room furniture is rearranged, zafus are placed on the floor, and they sit silently. In the kitchen, they eat fruit, drink tea, and catch up on each other's lives. She attends countless dharma talks given by Buddhist teachers. She subsequently trains with several Tibetan masters over prolonged periods. Her knowledge grows far deeper and her practice more mean-ingful.

A desire grows to share this knowledge and she valiantly tries to introduce this practice to her kids at a young age but they are skeptical. She takes her husband and children to a family program at a Buddhist center in Los Angeles and after meditating for two minutes, her seven-year-old son turns to his father and asks, How long do I have to pretend someone stole my brain?

She volunteers at the Boys & Girls Club, devising games for children through which they can learn meditation. No one has done that before. She establishes an organization called Inner Kids that is dedicated to bringing contemplative practice to schools. She begins to train adults to teach children how to meditate, first locally, then nationally, then internationally. She publishes two books on the subject which are both translated into ten languages. Her work merges with what becomes known as the secular mindfulness movement and children are exposed to these techniques in schools around the world. She is recognized as a pioneer in children's meditation, gets interviewed by newspapers and web publications, on radio shows and podcasts. Strangers approach her, seeking wisdom. She feels good about it but also finds it funny when people perceive her to be a quasi-guru. She still identifies more with apprehensive young parents than with wise elders. Back in her college theater major days, she could not have imagined a story with a plot like this. And neither could I when I married her.

Fade to black.

\* \* \*

Enemas have always been a mystery to me. Like the moons of Saturn, I never gave them much thought. What kind of person thinks about enemas who isn't in that business? Doctors, nurses, fetishists; and we will not discuss those proclivities here. Your average person is not troubled by stray thoughts of flooded colons.

The previous summer Susan showed me an article in a health magazine by a woman who claimed to have had her breast cancer cured by Dr. Nicholas Gonzalez using nothing more than a combination of diet, vitamins, supplements, and coffee enemas. When I learned this last detail, I informed her that it is a good thing that after swearing off caffeine we didn't throw out the cappuccino maker. It was always my belief that if I could return to a level playing field, get rid of the cancer, I could keep it from coming back by attacking the root cause. Traditional practitioners refuse to see past the symptoms but the problem is at once both simpler and more complex than that. Why should one person's immune system be able to fight it off when another person is not so lucky? Perhaps cancer grows in bad soil. Perhaps if the soil is made healthy, bad flowers will not return.

The poetry of Charles Baudelaire takes on new meaning: *Les fleurs du mal.*

Coffee enemas? *Pourquoi pas?*

We track Dr. Gonzales down and it turns out he's in New York City. He agrees to meet with me.

I've never done anything like this in my life.

Susan and I are ushered into his office in a quiet neighborhood in the East 30s, not far from the NYU hospital where I spent the past eight months being obliterated by chemotherapy, and where before I had masturbated into a cup. It's like I am committing medical adultery and if Dr. Speyer finds out he will cast me into the wilderness. Dr. Gonzalez sits behind a large desk. He is fifty years old but with his unlined face and full head of thick brown hair looks thirty-five. Diminutive with a puckish mien, friendly, conversational, and passionate about his treatment. We listen intently as he tells us he attended Brown University and Cornell Medical College before discovering the work of Dr. William Kelley, a man who had trained as a dentist and orthodontist. My heart sinks a little. Dentist and orthodontist? Please, no. But I have vowed to be open to new modes not just of thinking but of being so I tamp down my concerns, my tendency to judgment, and my most basic

instincts and stay focused. He was talking about Dr. Kelley—
Dr. Kelley was shoved brusquely into the spotlight when he
cared for the movie star Steve McQueen. It did not end well
for Steve McQueen. I quickly push *that* thought aside. The
regimen Kelley developed was based on the use of pancreatic
enzymes and this became the cornerstone for the work of Dr.
Gonzalez.

The debate about the efficacy of alternative procedures is as
old as medicine itself and I do not intend to engage in it here.
George Washington's doctors bled him on his deathbed. Leeches
were a mainstream means of treatment not that long ago and are
still employed in more adventurous precincts. I suspect in the not
too distant future people will look back on chemotherapy and
radiation with a jaundiced eye. This is not to say all alternative
therapies are inherently good. Obviously, they're not. But since
the mainstream medical establishment offers only "Good luck!"
I choose to be open to the universe. Not open like the village
idiot, mind you. I'm engaging in due diligence and counting on
my own discernment. That the Gonzalez treatment is based on
the work of an orthodontist means nothing. Well, not *nothing*. I
would prefer it were otherwise, a chemist or biologist would be
slightly less comical and easier to defend. But orthodontist it is
and I choose to be at peace with that. Charles Darwin was not
even trained as a scientist. And it's already been decided that I'm
going to do *something*.

I assume Dr. Gonzalez will immediately put me on a diet of
brown rice and mung beans because everyone knows a macrobiotic diet is the healthiest way to eat. He quickly corrects this
misapprehension and informs me that radical vegetarian diets
are only appropriate for people with "hard tumor" cancers—
these would be the classics: lung, breast, pancreatic, et al. For
soft tumor cancers like leukemia or lymphoma (go team!), Dr.
Gonzalez maintains the proper diet is one high in protein, and
animal fat, and heavy on red meat.

*Heavy on red meat?*

I'm genuinely shocked. This is when Dr. Gonzalez tells me about the Eskimos.

"The Eskimos had virtually no heart disease or cancer in their communities," he says. "Most of their diet consisted of whale meat, which is remarkably fatty. When they gradually switched to the white man's diet, their cancer and heart disease rates skyrocketed."

Who knew? I'm further amazed when he tells me a vegetarian diet creates a high alkaline environment in which soft tumors flourish. He is convinced that simply cutting my intake of red meat contributed to the lymphoma. I don't believe I caused my own illness, but I take his point.

I ask him what kind of success rate he's had with lymphoma patients, and he assures me it's quite high. "I was treating this one patient," Dr. Gonzalez says. "The man was not psychologically able to handle the red meat diet so he checked himself into a clinic where they placed him on a vegetarian diet."

"What happened?" I ask.

"His lymphoma exploded."

Salad: the silent assassin. Have I eaten my last arugula leaf?

This is all highly unsettling because virtually *all* the reading I've done suggests that the best way to prevent cancer is with a vegetarian diet. This community laughs at red meat. Dr. Gonzalez points out that when I ate red meat regularly I was always healthy. At first, I find the reasoning a tad facile. Then I think about it and realize that if I'm going to do this, I need to "commit to the bit," as they say in comedy. The luxury of remission allows me to take this step.

He examines me, then takes a lock of my hair to send to the lab for analysis. Hair analysis is a controversial diagnostic tool. Dr. Gonzalez claims that every element in the body is present in the hair and from this test he can determine—insofar as vitamins and enzymes are concerned—exactly how the soup should be seasoned. We make a second appointment to see him in a few weeks at which point he will prescribe an individual program. I don't want to wait a couple of weeks, my engine is revving, but there's no choice.

The low note in the distance, recurrence, persists. I must stop thinking about death all the time, about *time* all the time. The illness has increased my appreciation of so many things but the shroud it has cast can be unbearable. I tell myself that even if the cancer does recur, new therapies are being developed at an exponential rate. The Gonzalez treatment sounds promising. If nothing else, it will give me something on which to concentrate my palpitating energy.

I listen to tapes of lectures given by Dr. Gonzalez. Evangelical in his convictions, his enthusiasm bursts through the speakers. His theories convince me that by putting myself in his care, I am making the right decision. In hurried cadences, he claims the protocol creates a massive healing event in the body. Whereas the chemotherapists are adept at killing cells, the Gonzalez program pummels your cell structure, regenerating the entire system in the process.

Two weeks slow-walk by and we see Dr. Gonzales again. At the second appointment, he guides us through the regimen. Briefly: between vitamins and pancreatic enzymes I will be taking over a hundred pills a day at five different times. I will also take a dose at 3:00 A.M. so sleeping through the night is over.

Then Dr. Gonzalez holds up an enema bag. It looks like a sight gag, something you'd buy in a novelty shop, the medical equivalent of a whoopee cushion. Susan has to bite her lip to keep from dissolving into a fit of hysteria. To me, however, it is the holy chalice, the container for the elixir of life. Dr. Gonzales informs me I will do four coffee enemas a day, two in the morning and two in the afternoon.

Excuse me? *Four* enemas? Per day?

The theory behind the coffee enemas is this: the pancreatic enzymes break down the cancer cells that are still floating around in the body and the coffee hyper-activates the liver, causing it to flush out the detritus. In addition to the vitamins, enzymes, and coffee enemas, there is an even more intensive liver flush that involves Epsom salts, whipping cream, olive oil, berries, a gallon of apple juice, and Bentonite, a substance that bears a remarkable resemblance to liquid cement. Then there is something called the Clean Sweep, a sandblasting of the entire intestinal tract, the results of which allow for the vitamins and enzymes to be absorbed more efficiently into the body. I am to have 5-7 servings of fatty red meat (yes, that's right, *fatty red meat*), all of which must be organic, each week. And this is to be washed down by no less than a quart of freshly squeezed organic carrot juice a day. None of this will be simple. As far as produce goes, our local health food store is unimpressive. And where do you find a steady supply of organic meat?

With all of the alternative treatments available, why am I choosing the Gonzalez protocol, which seems extreme? The extremity is the point. The radical nature of his approach is what I hunger for. It doesn't feel like a half-measure. It's not passive. There are tasks and measurable results in the form of ongoing scans. In committing to this, I feel like I have joined an elite circle.

Although the Gonzalez protocol sounds like it was devised by a CIA black site interrogator I am elated when we leave his office. I thrive on the idea of an assignment, and now I have one. While I have bumped against authority my entire life, to this I click my heels and salute. The Gonzalez regimen will be like following a particularly elaborate order. The procuring and the sorting of the pills, the buying and preparing of the organic food, the business with the coffee (also organic) will create form from the internal chaos. I will be a monk in the Abbey of Wellness, a warrior. Can I be a monk *and* a warrior?

*We will not flag or fail.*

And where do we go right after seeing Dr. Gonzalez? Why, to Dr. Speyer, of course; for my monthly examination. Overcoming my discomfort, I mention that I am seeing Dr. Gonzalez and he looks at me as if I've told him I am going to contact Winston Churchill at a séance. He is so dismissive that discussion is pointless. Dr. Speyer informs us he wants to do another scan in a month to see if there is any activity in my abdomen. If he finds a clambake going on down there, he will prescribe additional chemo. If that happens, I am not certain what I will do. What he's offering is temporary control of a problem he admits he can't cure. And yet his approach vanquished the tumors. Might these malignancies be plotting, diminished but not destroyed, and now reconstituting in preparation for a second horrific assault? Who knows? But now I am encouraged by Gonzalez who thinks I can prosper on his program and by reconstituting my system with the various purges, cleanses, and sweeps cure me, yes, that is correct, *cure me* of this disease.

When I next see Dr. Gonzales and mention the traditionalists consider themselves unable to cure low-grade lymphoma he tells me I'm not in that world anymore. Cancer represents authority and I am a revolutionary. The totalitarian state will be overthrown.

Despite the extremely daunting notion of having to follow a protocol that requires me to ingest exponentially more tablets and capsules than Ken Kesey and the Merry Pranksters took on their bus tour of North America, I am inspired. Although I recognize I will need to be cognizant of my intake every conscious hour, with time it will settle into a routine. Work for your health and you appreciate it that much more.

A lifelong carnivore, I salivate at the prospect of being turned loose on a diet of red meat. Unfortunately, the red meat must be organic and organic red meat is nearly impossible to find. We order half a cow, literally, from an organic farm in Michigan that Catie has tracked down. It arrives frozen, packed in coolers. We pick it up at the local airport on a cold, windy, early spring afternoon. That night I eat a steak for the first time in years. Susan cooks the slab of beef, seasons it, serves it with a baked potato and a side of green beans. The meat is so tough, cutting it I nearly sprain my wrist. I chew extensively before I dare swallow. Worry what damage I'm doing to my teeth. It's not marbled or in any way delicious. It does not even taste particularly good. This is far from the pleasurably carnivorous homecoming I expected. And I've committed to devouring an entire freezer cooler of the stuff. And another. Ad infinitum. Yet I'm thrilled.

I ask Dr. Gonzalez about meditation. He tells me that he doesn't recommend it for someone like me since it would raise my alkaline level and, as I have learned, lymphoma takes to a high alkaline environment like a dog to a summer lake.

To review:

Vegetarianism: bad. Meditation: bad. Fatty red meat: good.

Shibboleths are falling right and left. I'm confused. Dr. Gonzalez's mentor, Dr. William Kelley, was prohibited from operating a clinic in the United States and decamped to Mexico, which is where Steve McQueen found him. When a not particularly broad-minded relative heard I was being treated by Dr. Gonzalez, her subtle response was to imitate a duck: quack, quack, quack. Point taken. There are endless alternative cures for cancer around the world. Someone named John of God lives in Brazil and claims to remove patients' diseased guts without surgery. That seems a bit much; I won't be flying to Brazil. As for Gonzalez, his traditional training reassures me, as does his sunny east side office. His eccentric treatment can be framed as an extension of what I've been doing. But why do I need to keep doing anything? Why can't I just relax and enjoy remission like a normal person? Because it feels as if I've been released into the wild by Dr. Speyer and, like a house cat among the leopards, I'm on edge. There are sounds in the night. Did the branch just move or was that a large snake? A hunger pain feels like it might be stomach cancer, a tweaked knee a bone tumor. A person can drive themselves crazy. I need a touchstone, a shaman—albeit one with a degree from a prestigious medical school—to equip me for the struggle to survive physically and psychologically. I need to be given a plan that will allow me to face the Kierkegaardian moment with something more than a stupid look on my face. Worst-case scenario is that all of this accomplishes nothing. The point is, I'm *doing* something. And I don't have to do everything Dr. Gonzalez says. Perhaps I *will* meditate.

The pills arrive a few days later in a large box. Unpacking, I lay my future on the dining room table in Cold Spring. Thousands of pills, hundreds of glassine envelopes. The table looks like a pharmaceutical factory. Sorting the first week's supply: one of this kind, two of that, three of the other, all neatly placed in glassine envelopes, each one representing a single serving. The idea is to have each dose in an envelope so I can carry them around and pop them, regardless of where I happen to find myself. It is a bracing morning in late April and I am saving my life. The enzymes and vitamins run through my fingers like gambling chips. I am betting on Dr. Gonzalez, everything on red twenty-seven, spin the wheel.

Creating a one-week supply takes me an hour.

While I do this, I brew a pot of coffee I will not be drinking.

*Les fleurs du mal ne reviendront pas.*

* * *

It is with no small sense of foreboding that I proceed to the next step of the Gonzalez program. Coffee pot in hand, I nervously ascend to the bathroom I have commandeered as my World Health Headquarters/Cafe. I close the door behind me and take a deep breath. Then I unbutton and remove my shirt, pull off my jeans, step out of my underwear. I fold the clothes and place the pile on the rim of the bathtub. Naked, I am dressed for success. I have had the foresight to turn up the heat, so at least I'm not shivering as I prepare for this supremely undignified moment. Without giving away too much of my personal life—not that it isn't already a little late for that—I will tell you that I am not accustomed to having foreign objects inserted into my rectum. No one is telling gerbil jokes about me. I grew up in the age of rectal thermometers and as a young father am jealous every time a pediatrician takes my children's temperature by putting something in their ear for two seconds. As a child, I hated being sick since it meant my mother would be wielding her thermometer which swelled, in my mind, to the size of a baton whenever it got near me. And now I am meant to put eighteen inches of rubber tubing up there to be followed by an aromatic beverage.

All right, I think. Quit stalling.

I fill a clear plastic enema bag with lukewarm coffee from the stainless-steel pot and hang it from a doorknob. A towel is placed on the floor over the cold tiles. Then I slather the lube on the red tubing, lie down, and violate myself. Unclamping the tube, I recline on my left side and wait. And wait. But nothing happens. What is going on here? The coffee refuses to flow. Here I am lying on the floor with a rubber tube in my rectum, everything in suspended animation and, worst of all, bereft of reading material. After a moment of teeth-gnashing, it occurs to me that the problem might be gravity. Perhaps I have not hung the enema bag from a high enough altitude and that is impeding the coffee from cascading southward to its destination. Luckily the back of the bathroom door sports a peg from which to hang a towel. I remove the tube and place the enema bag up there. But—oh, god—I have forgotten to clamp the tube and suddenly coffee is gushing, rushing down like a caffeinated black mountain stream. In a moment, it has flooded the bathroom floor and a widening lake of warm organic coffee surrounds me. Cursing, dripping, I quickly clamp the tube. I have rarely been happier no one was observing me.

Thump Thump Thump—pounding on the door. Susan.

"Can you watch the kids? I need to go to the market."

My feet are wet, the towel soaked with coffee.

"Not now. Can you wait a little while?"

There is a long pause and then: "What's going on in there?"

"Nothing!"

"I heard you cursing. Are you all right?"

"Tip-top!"

"That coffee smells really strong."

"I know. I know—I'm okay. I'll see you when I'm done."

"What's it like?"

"What's what like?"

"Having all that coffee up your butt."

"Did you really just ask me that question?"

"Yes, I did."

"I'll tell you later."

"All right, good luck. I'll take the kids with me."

Mercifully, she retreats, leaving me alone on the battlefield.

I take the towel on which I have been lying and mop up the mess. The room smells like 8:00 A.M., every café in America. Ordinarily, this is pleasant but today less so. I place a clean towel on the floor. There is enough coffee in the pot to perform another enema, so I reload. Recline, reinsert. My diagnosis of gravity has proven correct and when the clamp is released the coffee cascades, filling my colon. The sensation is strange, this warmth emanating from the inside, a slight pressure on the interior wall of my intestines. It is not entirely unpleasant.

It is pleasing to have solved the engineering problem, but that feeling of satisfaction lasts for about five seconds at which point I am consumed with a desire to expel the coffee. My stomach hardens, as if by contracting my abdominal wall any involuntary action can be forestalled. I clench. I tense. I grit. For two nearly endless minutes—holding, holding, holding—at which point I dive for the toilet where the coffee rockets out with the force of a space capsule bursting through the Earth's atmosphere. By the time this effusion concludes, I am a popped balloon, inside out, collapsed. It feels as if one of my organs may have accidentally dislodged and slipped into the toilet. And yet the caffeine has provided me with a sudden buzz. A bizarre combination—I am hollow but perky.

As with most things that don't involve the handling of wild animals, the more you do them, the less difficult they are and performing this particular ritual quickly becomes second nature. Moreover, I stop viewing it as strange. Other people are another story: You're doing what with coffee? No one can believe it but my friends, none of whom have had to deal with cancer, treat me like a war veteran. I have gravitas. Nobody tells me I'm crazy to be doing this when, on the surface at least, it looks crazy. Because I have been to places they have not been, seen things they can only imagine and would frankly prefer not to. My experience with Stage 4 cancer gives me an earned authority so no one questions my decision, at least to my face. What they might say when I leave the room can only be surmised. That is another story entirely. In earshot of everyone who learns of this regimen, I receive nothing but support. And when I begin to explain the theory behind the coffee deployment, they listen and it becomes slightly less funny, although not entirely lacking in comedy because when they conjure the visual—

Now it's just a particularly colorful strand in the fabric of my existence.

Each day I wake up, swallow pills, pulp ten carrots and drink the juice, do two coffee enemas. Then I eat breakfast and make for my Cold Spring home office which is adjacent to my World Health Headquarters. There I spend the morning, taking breaks, during which I consume more pills. I eat lunch and take more pills. Then I pulp another ten carrots, drink the juice, and do a pair of mid-afternoon enemas. More pills, dinner, still more pills, spend time with my family in the evening, even more pills, go to sleep, wake up in the middle of the night for yes, more pills, then get up and repeat the process. I have no idea how anyone who does not work at home can do this. Rather than feeling put upon, I feel extremely fortunate.

I rarely skip a dosage of pills, but appointments will occasionally cause me to miss an enema. And yes, it feels strange to type that last sentence. Given my rate of pill consumption, this deviation is allowable. At a child's birthday party, or visiting in-laws, or having lunch with a friend in the city, I am calculating when I will be able to do the next enema. When I fly to California for business meetings, the enema kit is packed: bag, tube, organic coffee, stainless steel coffee pot.

I am reclining on a bathroom floor, having grown accustomed to the view, in a fancy Marina Del Rey hotel room that some studio is springing for. It's enema time. Perk, pour, spread the towel, lie down, insert, relax. I am perusing a magazine when the phone rings—it's a producer who has recently purchased one of my screenplays, a cause for momentary celebration which has already dissipated. Before he can massacre it (which he will proceed to do), there are notes he'd like to share. I don't want to hear his niggling notes but that's the job and I have no choice. The producer, a young gasbag whose abrasiveness is unmitigated by his arrogance, is a fan of the Socratic method since it allows him to accentuate the power dynamic, so he asks me a lot of questions intended to solicit answers he already knows in what is more of a primate dominance demonstration than what is known as a "notes call." Were he in the room I'd be tempted to wrap the enema tube around his neck and pull it until his eyes pop but because I am now slouching toward enlightenment I politely listen as he prattles on. And while he prattles, I float out of my body and observe my naked form from the perspective of the bathroom ceiling, prostrate on the tile floor, colon filled to the brim with warm coffee, enduring the producer's annoying personality, and I am looking down on the luckiest man in the world.

\* \* \*

The sense of heightened anxiety I lived with during that post-treatment period was a constant companion. Every shower was an opportunity to examine my armpits, my groin, my neck, searching for swelling. Vitamins and supplements by the handful. The coffee routine. Coruscating cleanses. Skin brushing. Embracing Horse. My will to live was the animating principle that propelled me from moment to moment and only when I slept was there respite. While this was going on, my friend Leonard suffered an emotional collapse and checked into a psychiatric facility north of the city. He had lost his radio gig interviewing comedians, and his coping mechanisms, such as they were, had ceased to function. He was feeling suicidal and his wife Emily had committed him. Years earlier, before we knew each other, a similar crisis had played out. I was optimistic that he would pull himself together.

It was the day before Easter when I went to visit him. On the drive I thought about the times we had spent together cogitating on the meaning of it all, the rolling laughs exalted and inane. When he opened the door of the comedy world, it set me on a path from which I had never strayed. To know he was hurting and in danger was upsetting and there was nothing to do but go and be present. Never having been to a mental hospital, I experienced a sense of trepidation and nervousness driving on to the grounds. Visions of austere staff, oppressive security protocols, patients feeble or agitated. But the facility felt more like a progressive liberal arts college. A series of inviting, humanely scaled buildings on a verdant campus. It was easy to imagine a professor of Gender Theory strolling over the greensward, books tucked under her arm, frisbees sailing overhead. No metal bars, no attendants in hospital whites.

I signed in and after a few minutes Leonard appeared in street clothes looking entirely himself, if a little thinner.

"Babe," he said when he saw me.

"Babe," I echoed.

To my relief, he smiled. When we embraced his bones felt birdlike, delicate. He led me to his residence, a two-story, brown, shingled building. His spartan room was on the first floor. A bed, a chair, a desk. All immaculate. He sat on the bed and I settled into the chair. The door remained open, a hard and fast rule.

"So," I said, "what are *you* doing here?" He laughed.

We chatted as if we were drinking coffee in the old Prince Street apartment. Leonard joked and complained about his depression as if it were an unreliable acquaintance who had showed up to borrow money and I about the difficulty of the holidays. The previous evening Susan had announced that she wanted to take Allegra to Easter services. After more than a year of meditation, tai chi, and learning to let go, my reaction to this declaration reflected none of that.

"I know how silly it is to be threatened by Susan's virtually secular take on Easter—"

"Eggs and rabbits," Leonard said.

"But if my kid goes to an Easter service I'll feel like a traitor to the Jews."

"This Jew doesn't care," Leonard assured me.

"Yeah, but rather than it be about the subtle cultivation of our children's spiritual lives my entire psyche is ruled by these primitive impulses that block any movement toward true metaphysical development, whatever that's supposed to look like."

"You should take your daughter to a Hasidic reading room," Leonard said, and launched into a bit about the ushers at the synagogue in which he had grown up who refused to interrupt their elaborate prayer rituals while seating the congregants, complete with voices and gestures; a clatter of chanted Hebrew in which the only two recognizable words were *Mrs. Feigenbaum*, the woman presumably being shown to her pew. It would have killed in a club.

When I finished laughing, I explored my troubles in great detail, my insuperable tribal identity, and failure to attain a sliver of illumination, as Leonard listened attentively. All of this served up while the poor guy was recovering from a nervous breakdown. But I don't think he minded. Leonard seemed to enjoy focusing on someone else's tribulations.

We spent two hours together that afternoon. I did not know much about depression at the time and, while sympathetic to his predicament, the irony that he had been contemplating suicide when I would have given anything within my power for more life was not lost on me.

A week later Leonard was discharged and we saw each other regularly until I moved to California. Years passed and then Emily died unexpectedly. She was sixty-six. The next time I was back in New York, I went to visit him. It had been a while since we had seen each other and I was concerned about the toll grief would take on the eggshell of his psyche. We were seated in his spacious Upper West Side living room on the 11th floor of a pre-war building. I remembered parties and dinners here. A warm place, filled with art and life, quiet now.

"How are you doing?"

"Don't worry," he said. "I'm not going to kill myself."

I returned to Los Angeles. My son was making plans to

spend a year at a school in Manhattan and needed an afford-able place to live. I thought of Leonard rattling around that apartment and whether he might want a young roommate. The idea came to nothing.

The following winter, haunted by his father's suicide, and unable to imagine a desirable future for himself, Leonard jumped from the roof of the building where he had lived for twenty years with Emily. Separated by a continent we had drifted apart, but I found myself gutted upon hearing the news. There were pangs of guilt about not staying in closer touch. Was there anything else I could have done? The vanity in that question provides the answer. His suffering was ineluctable and it was impossible to judge him for the path he had chosen.

My friend Judy knew Leonard from the old days and the following week the two of us sat shiva at a rib joint on Ventura Boulevard where we toasted his memory and recalled some of the jokes he loved to tell. Like this one:

A man falls from a twelve-story building. Guy at a sixth floor window yells, How's it going? And the falling man says, So far, so good.

\* \* \*

I accompany Dad to *his* oncologist. How infinitely better it would be if I were accompanying him to his numismatist, but no, it's an oncologist. His low-grade lymphoma has returned but the doctor is not going to treat it yet. They perform a bone marrow extraction on him, a procedure with which he is as familiar as I. Allegra has the chicken pox now. I need to keep my distance from the virus but the house is big enough so this is possible.

I finish my first fifteen-day Gonzalez vitamin/enzyme treatment and begin a five-day clean sweep. It is like drinking liquid cardboard several times a day. This creates pristine intestines with nothing left to impede the absorbing of the vitamins. I am in the middle of the clean sweep when I go back to NYU Medical Center for a scan. When I get home, I pray. Yes, that's right. I keep with it. For months, I've ended each qigong session with a prayer of thanks but recently I've been praying independently of the qigong. Out loud. I've been talking to God out loud, or some version of the idea of God—my religiosity waxes and wanes hourly. I'm "praying" several times a day this spring. For help, courage, protection of my family. I don't know if my vision of God will ever solidify or will it exist in a constant state of becoming. But I don't let that stop me. I've also stopped telling God to go fuck Himself.

At this new stage of life, it would be unbecoming.

Here is my current prayer:

*Dear God OR the random series of events that created music and jokes and beer and wine and Indian food and books and movies and Bangkok and Joshua Tree National Park and worn-in sneakers and basketball and the Hudson River at sunset as seen from Lower Manhattan, the beach at Montauk at sunrise, cheeseburgers, steamed clams at a seaside shack and modern art and modern medicine and pancreatic enzymes: thank you for the things in life that bring me pleasure, fulfillment and joy, especially my kids. Thank you for the true heart of my wife. Thank you for the wherewithal to explore the options available to me and Writers Guild health insurance. Thank you for helping me to thrive again. Thank you for this day. Thank you for life. As Charles Dickens wrote in another context: please, sir, may I have some more? Amen.*

The lively internal dialogue continues. I get the results of the full-body scan. Completely clean.

But the new diet and the coffee routine have a strange effect. I begin to lose weight. Five pounds, then ten, fifteen, twenty. One day I am walking in our house and—*ping*, I hear the soft sound of gold delicately striking wood. My wedding ring has slipped from my finger. I have accidentally dropped from 183 pounds to 158. This is not weight I can afford to lose. Like the woman from the health food store, I am a wraith. Terrified that I am disappearing.

\* \* \*

It turns out that thinking about the afterlife, unless someone is paying you, is a waste of precious time. The Egyptians, the Jews, Christians, Buddhists, Muslims, and Hindus? All of their projections are right, every one of them. How can this be so? Because they function as a collective salve to the wound of the unanswerable question. The wound is painful and it never heals. You learn to live with it.

\* \* \*

My practice evolves. Between 6:00 and 6:30 A.M., I get up and do the coffee routine. There is an hour of qigong then a breakfast of yogurt and nuts. If the way I feel is any indication, the Gonzalez program is working. After a year of wild zigzags, life is in an easier flow. I spend the day at my desk writing. Clouds gather and when they inevitably fray the sun beams down on the highland hills, golden and strong. I am still orange from all the beta carotene in the carrot juice, a minor drawback. I don't *like* being orange. Or skin and bones.

I pick up my appointment calendar for the past year, the hell year. Each month appears on the right side of the book as a grid of days. On the left side is a reproduction of a painting. The painting for this month is *Birthday* by Marc Chagall. It depicts a young woman in profile. Pitched forward at a sixty-degree angle, she is standing near a vanity holding a bouquet of flowers. A young man hovers above her, floating on his back. His head curls over in a serpentine way and he is about to kiss her.

Under the day's date I have written: To Miss Connie's.

We take Allegra to visit her nursery school. As she lets go of our hands and wanders off to explore, there's a lump in my throat. Gabe, buoyant, is nearly crawling. When Susan was pregnant, I was so preoccupied I barely noticed. Now that he is here, he fascinates me, laughing pure baby laughs.

This health regimen, vitamins, enzymes, enemas—continues for a year. Then another. It becomes the foundation and beams of my life. What holds up the house. My strength returns. My hair grows back. The weight I precipitously lost slowly returns. It's not easy to find organic food in the Hudson Valley but I am a hard-bitten sleuth in my efforts to track it down. At Thanksgiving Dad manages to find an organic turkey. As a party trick, I take thirty pills at once. I play with my kids every day, shoot videos of all the cornball things: first steps, first day of school, first Halloween costume. Susan transitions back from caretaker to wife. To my indescribable relief, I have not betrayed her by dying. I do another scan and it's as clean as the one before. And so is the next one. And the one after that. And so on.

# EPILOGUE

For five years, I rigidly followed the Gonzalez program. At that point I had performed nearly five thousand coffee enemas, entire contents of untold chain franchises sluicing through my system, and ingested scores of thousands of vitamins and enzymes. Traditionally, the five-year mark is when a person goes from "in remission" to "cured" and although I don't subscribe to all the tenets of traditional treatment, five years seems like a reasonable metric. I ratcheted down my adherence to the regimen and now do a fraction of what I did back then. For a while this winding down was slightly nervous-making. But one of the truisms about having children is that they allow you to stop thinking so much about yourself and since mine were (a) a toddler and (b) in utero when this started, it wasn't that difficult to turn my focus outward. The bedlam of our house made self-obsession an ongoing challenge.

Occasionally the kids would pipe down or sleep and that would be when meditation might happen. Although I don't consider myself religious, I still pray occasionally, usually in thanks, never in supplication. It's not like anyone's listening, but the activity calms and can't hurt. Atheists are as dogmatic as fundamentalists and I have learned to distrust all received wisdom.

Many friends from that time are still in my life but not all of them. Max left New York City and moved to the Pacific Northwest where he works as a life coach. He resumed writing fiction, creating a character based on himself called the Quill, a Zen Buddhist Jew who roams Seattle "snacking on bagel chips and seeking satori." A collection of offbeat stories, *Tales of the Quill*, was first-rate and I tried to help get them published, with no luck.

When I was in the Mojave Desert staying at the Inn at Twenty-Nine Palms and polishing the manuscript of a novel we had a phone call. One of the most articulate and passionate people I've ever known, Max had a Fidel Castro-like ability to hold the floor while on the phone. One time he was so carried away by one of his monologues that I dropped the receiver on my desk, walked down the hall to take care of some business and returned a few minutes later. When I pressed the phone back to my ear he was volubly chattering away, oblivious to my absence. In the desert on this day, that is not what happened.

It was late on a temperate afternoon and I was smoking a cigar for the nicotine as I marked up pages with red ink. The conversation turned to Obama who at the time was in his first term. My friend, who was a proponent of spiritual awakening and inordinately proud of his own, displayed what I took to be an irrational contempt for the president. No president is above criticism of course, and Obama had his flaws, but Max's opinion seemed to come from somewhere beyond politics. Our exchange began to heat up, and then heat up some more, and Max told me in complete seriousness that I was "radically unenlightened," something I have never forgotten, because it's probably the most purely Buddhist insult anyone has ever invented. While it sounds as if it were meant as a gag, he was deadly serious. It was the most wounding thing, to Max's way of thinking, that he could summon.

But, but, but—

This is someone who was deeply present in the hour of my distress. The Chinese medicine he introduced me to may have been chimerical but the tai chi and qigong heightened my focus and were both a physical and psychological boon. When I was sick, he looked me in the eye. Not everyone did. Friendship should not be complicated, and yet—

I heard from Max when Leonard died. We hadn't spoken in the years since our fiery exchange and that phone call had been a disaster. What is the etiquette when a guy with whom you're no longer on speaking terms calls you out of the blue to discuss the suicide of someone you both loved?

Although we both were experiencing deep sadness our conversation was brief.

The chasm was not bridged.

I wished him well.

After four years in the Hudson Valley we moved to California. Los Angeles with a family turned out to be a far better fit. For all of its unpredictable fires, predictable droughts, mind-bending traffic, occasionally crusty air, June gloom, punishing heat, and vast downtown homeless encampment, there is kayaking at dawn on the Los Angeles River, hiking in the mountains and the desert, Disney Hall and the Los Angeles Philharmonic playing a new John Adams piece, dinners with friends in Little India, food trucks on Wilshire Boulevard that sell delicious Korean tacos, Clipper games at the Staples Center, Lucinda Williams at the Troubadour, the Los Angeles Times Book Festival and the Los Angeles Review of Books, hidden Chinatown galleries that show challenging work by emerging artists and the classical profusion of the Getty Villa, stolen glimpses of cerulean Hockney pools in the Hollywood Hills, the scent of bougainvillea spilling over the white stucco walls of a mission-style house in Silver Lake, the limitless western view from the Santa Monica cliffs high above the ocean booming in the violet distance; it's the place where our children grew up.

We never went back to Repro.

For the past twenty-five years I have thought about death more than most people my age. Like a guest that has arrived too early for a dinner party, its presence caught me unprepared. And like an early party guest, it could not be told to come back later. Death made itself at home, mixed a drink and whispered, breath on my neck, words obscure—*I'm sorry, what's that, I didn't quite catch what you said*—but then unexpectedly packed up and slipped away, leaving me trembling with an awareness I did not previously possess. Friends my age, the age of marriage and children and chasing careers, knew the facts, the diagnosis, treatment, recovery, but they had not felt the cold breath. Perhaps they noticed the shadow in my eyes. It was not something anyone wanted to talk about.

My friend Jeff was a screenwriter and we came up in the business together. His wife was a lawyer and they had two kids. We were leading parallel lives. While I was still being treated, he showed me a screenplay he had written where a secondary character had lymphoma and it was handled like a joke. Fair enough, but at the time it made me uncomfortable because Jeff was healthy and I was not. A few years later, he got cancer and died. I wish that was a joke.

Humans are divided from animals by many things but cognizance of our impending non-being is perhaps the most salient one. While it's natural to ignore this aspect of our brief existence, and most do, that option was foreclosed to me. Once I was afforded the joy of survival, rather than just quickly putting the experience behind me and returning to my pre-sickness state of willfully ignorant bliss, the vivid awareness remained prominent in my psyche. I had psychological progeria, which is to say that in my head I became old early. Not superannuated in that risk-averse, cantankerous, world-has-gone-to-shit sense, but in the way that I *knew* what it was like to feel the nearness of oblivion. Standing at the edge, I had peered over.

This awareness affected my professional choices. In writing movies or television, the main idea is to get paid. Obviously, you want the work to be high quality, but if this is how you make your living, money must change hands. The studio has to believe your script, when produced, is going to allow them to make a profit. My years in the screenwriting trenches had left me with a desire to explore stories that were not necessarily going to set cash registers ringing. If I wanted to fulfill my earliest ambitions, there was work to be done and I had been granted a felt sense of the increasingly limited time in which to accomplish it. From my early addiction to the Hardy Boys mysteries, I have always been drawn to the novel and in 2005 I published my first, *The Bones*. My fifth, *The Hazards of Good Fortune*, came out last year. It's been my immense good luck to receive positive reviews and sell movie or television rights to all of them. They've been translated into foreign languages. Along the way I taught fiction writing in Los Angeles. Several of my former students have now published well-received novels.

Since reading Richard Halliburton's travel classic *The Royal Road to Romance* when I was in college, I've wanted to circumnavigate the world and although I haven't quite managed that feat, Susan and I have visited nearly forty countries. In Indonesia, we climbed to the top of Borobudur, the world's oldest Buddhist temple complex, witnessed the Vietnamese flag raised at dawn in front of Ho Chi Minh's tomb in Hanoi, walked the Old City of Jerusalem, rafted the Grand Canyon, crawled through the Turkish cave city of Cappadocia. In Paris, I've participated in literary festivals and appeared on panels with authors far more famous (although it's certain I'm the only one who has worked with both Rodney Dangerfield *and* Chloe Sevigny). Last year I drove back and forth across America for the third time.

I'm not racing but I keep moving.

Why was there no recurrence? Asking that question makes me slightly nervous, which proves that, for all my attempts at self-improvement, even today I am hardly a model of perfect equanimity. The writing of this book was an exercise in getting me to finally consider what happened, put my experience in some kind of perspective, give form to it and allow me to see if it might somehow be useful to anyone else. So, can the past quarter century of good health be attributed to the Gonzalez program? Again, like the efficacy of prayer, who knows? There are a great many people who would like to think so.

I have been asked many times what I would do if I was ever again diagnosed with cancer. Would I have chemotherapy and radiation or would I eschew traditional treatment and go straight to an alternative regimen? There was a firm answer to that in the years immediately following my diagnosis but, as with all things, my response today would be more nuanced. Now I can say that the course of treatment would depend on what I was dealing with and the nature of the prognosis. The unavoidable fact, the *truth*: traditional medicine obliterated my cancer. Traditional medicine also assured me it would come back. In this case, one out of two was not a bad average. Although I began my alternative regimen with an I'll show them attitude, today I am anything but smug regarding the traditionalists being wrong about recurrence. I am only grateful they were right about how to treat it.

Following a demanding protocol provided a structure on to which I could hang my hopes, and hope is a commodity that needs a place to hang, to be treated tenderly and succored. For the discouraged and fearful, it is an element as essential as hydrogen and oxygen. Does everyone have the same result with the Gonzalez program? Sadly, no. I was fortunate. But there are many other patients of Dr. Gonzalez out there that are survivors, too.

Everyone who took junior high school science knows that for a hypothesis to be valid, the experiment must be repeatable in identical circumstances by anyone. Unfortunately, treating cancer is more complicated than a junior high school science project. Since none of us are identical on a cellular level, treatment of some diseases can be achingly difficult to predict. To this day, I have never asked Dr. Speyer to tell me the results of the clinical trial. I am healthy. I hope the other patients in the trial are, too.

It's not for me to give advice to anyone who finds themselves in a similar straits, unless I'm asked, in which case I'll talk your ear off. Prayer, herbs, crystals (wait, no, *not* crystals)—perhaps these things work for some people. Enzymes, vitamins, and coffee enemas can work, too. Or not. Some are saved by chemotherapy, others die. Answers are elusive. Luck is essential. When I am asked by anyone what kind of treatment they should pursue after they've been diagnosed with cancer, here is what I say: make a choice and believe in it. That is all you can do.

Some people will advise you to keep laughing. Feel free to decline. Or you can keep laughing. There's no cure for comedy.

And my health? There were some difficulties having to do with a severely compromised immune system and the havoc caused by the chemotherapy. I developed shingles, and ear infections so virulent they necessitated emergency room visits. Doctors treated the ear infections with antibiotics. It was only when I began to see a homeopath that they ceased. Again, that is not an endorsement of homeopathy. Some friends and relatives have tried it with no luck at all. Others have had remarkably positive results.

The only lesson I am not hesitant to impart from my experience is that we must not be afraid of the new.

Take risks, but be a little circumspect, too.

Don't let anyone else make choices for you.

Advocate for yourself.

Above all: always consider.

Are these words the younger version of me might have written? Likely not. Those probably would have been just as well-meaning but would have strained for laughs. The uncomfortable truth is that into my thirties I remained a bit of a calf. I'm not proud of that and don't make excuses for it. Life knocked me sideways but I took notes so it wasn't for nothing.

As someone on the receiving end of a lot of well-meaning speeches, I learned what to do when a friend finds out they're sick. Many people told me a lot of things and I can barely recall a word. Because most of the words don't mean anything. Yes, they have their familiar dictionary definitions, but in this kind of drama, words are just sounds that float like dust motes in a shaft of light before dissolving into nothingness.

Only presence has meaning. You remember who was there.

After a four-decade run, my father folded his business. He eventually married a woman closer to his own age and significantly less problematic. He settled into retirement and continued on his autodidactic path. As a grandfather, he was sublime. In 2011, he died and we buried him next to my mother, presumably facing the right direction.

My brother Drew trained as a yoga teacher and taught yoga to cancer patients at Memorial Sloan Kettering for ten years. He is now retired and lives in Connecticut.

When we moved to California, Susan put in an organic garden and grows tomatoes, cucumbers, broccolini, bok choy, zucchini, eggplant, lettuce, watermelon, snap peas, beans, peppers from which she makes sought-after hot sauce, and a panoply of flowers that she cuts and arranges in vases around the house. She continues to teach internationally and to write books and articles.

Right now, I am as healthy as someone my age can reasonably expect to be. For years I walked our dogs in the Santa Monica Mountains every day either at sunrise or sunset and did this until they were too old to go on walks. I drove the kids to school and sports practices and music lessons until they went off to college. They graduated and are now fully-fledged adults. Both are thriving. You will have to ask them for more specific details of their lives. Not long ago, I transferred all of our home videos, hours and hours, to a digital format. We haven't watched a single one.

When I am stuck in traffic, or have a frustrating moment in my work, or find myself in a quandary that might have loomed large at one point, one where things are not going exactly as I like, I can usually step back and appreciate that I'm here to experience it in the first place. Not always, I hasten to add. There are times I even forget what I went through, what I nearly lost. But never for long, and when I remember I'm always slightly abashed at having forgotten. I am more patient now, more prone to observe my thought process before acting.

Mostly.

Have I reached some kind of personal earthly exaltation where I exist on a level of consciousness others should strive to attain?

No.

I still can't carry a tune and remain hungry for experience.


So—

I am alone at a white-topped round table seated in a wicker chair. Birds flit over the temple adjacent to the ghat that inclines from Ahilya Fort in Maheshwar, India. Yes, India. Please don't judge me. I haven't become a Hindu or Buddhist and still have no claim to enlightenment.

Although the sun is low in the west, the temperature is vindaloo. A late afternoon breeze riffles the pages in my notebook. Sounds of boat engines and youthful voices drift up from the Narmada River. This is the violet hour when boatmen take tourists in longboats to the small temple on an island in the river that Hindus believe is the actual center of the world. A worker sweeps the terrace.

Descending the ghat I pass an elaborate temple complex. A few beggars, a goat, a gaggle of teenage girls in colorful saris, and boatmen looking for business. There are nine idle boats now and two on the river. A school of boys are swimming in the brown water. I sit on one of the steps to take in the panorama.

The Narmada is magnificent, the kind of river that inspired those who beheld it to think in mythic language, and it's wide where it flows past Maheshwar. Along the far shore the shapes of trees are reflected on the surface. The wooden boats are painted yellow, white, blue, green in various combinations, all pleasing to the eye. A man in an orange baseball cap hawks fruit from a round silver tray displayed on a wicker stand. A woman in a sari balancing a large bowl on her head, the contents wrapped in plastic, descends the ghat and passes to my left. Above and to my right a group of young girls call to me from a parapet and wave. There are no other westerners. A brown goat ambles east along the shoreline. Young Indians pose for pictures, boys in western dress, girls in a mixture of traditional and modern. The concrete has retained so much heat, it feels like my legs are hovering over a low flame. A group of women in wildly colored saris float down the steps like human confetti. In the river, a boy is taking his cow for a swim. Fish leap in the water. Yesterday Susan and I rode a longboat and now I see our boatman talking to the fruit vender with the orange baseball cap. A small brown goat passes two feet from me. The sun ceases to give off intense heat but now there are more boys in the river. The woman with the basket on her head sets up shop. No one buys anything from her or Orange Cap. A tourist boat motors along the dock but remains offshore. The boatman cuts the engine to allow his passengers to enjoy the view of the temple and ramparts. Some who pass ignore me, others say hello. No one is unfriendly or tries to sell me anything. The sun is hidden behind a few clouds now, almost at the horizon, and a soft gray light hangs over the river. A flock of small birds take wing in crazy, chaotic flight, an evening constitutional before turning in. The saturated colors of the saris dim in the gloaming. A humpbacked old woman with a cane greets me as she navigates down the steps. Orange Cap lights a mosquito coil on his fruit tray, a sweet pleasing smell. At last, some of the sari ladies buy fruit. A cow swims past, only her eyes visible above the water line. The lights above the parapet are illuminated as the birds continue to swoop through the temple arches. The evening awaits.

As I climb the steps an Indian woman asks if I will take her picture. Younger than me, but not young, she is alone and I comply, framing her with the river in the background. When I hand the camera back so she can see what I've done, she gazes at the image and says, It's good enough.

Time to pack; there are other towns to see.

In Varanasi we watch the mourners burn their dead.


END
Los Angeles, 2019

## Acknowledgments

I want to thank Anton Chekhov and his translators Richard Pevear and Larissa Volokhonsky. It was in their translation of his story *The Black Monk* that I chanced upon the phrase "a kingdom of tender colors." I thought it would make a fine title for this book.

Nearly all of the nurses, technicians, and doctors I encountered performed their tasks with admirable professionalism and kindness. Beth Taubes, aka Beth the Nurse, who ably led me through the wilderness of chemotherapy, needs to be singled out.

Among the many healthcare professionals deserving of recognition, Dr. James Speyer and Dr. Nicholas Gonzalez are in a special class. It is not hyperbole to say that I don't know if I would be alive today without them. Both are talented doctors and compassionate men, healers in the truest sense. Dr. Speyer was there in my darkest hour. I am deeply appreciative of his guidance and support during that time. Dr. Gonzalez provided hope and a renewed sense of the future when my future looked uncertain. But what was most impressive about these men, and what I value at the deepest level, is how much they cared. Never did I feel like just another patient.

I'm grateful to Tom Lutz, Diana Wagman, and Drew Greenland who read early versions of the text. When I sat down in a coffeeshop with Dinah Lenney, who took the time to discuss what was then a ten-year-old project of mine that had been stashed in a drawer, I left with an idea of how I might reapproach the material.

It has been my pleasure over many years now to be represented by the discerning, perceptive, and wise agents Henry Dunow and Sylvie Rabineau. Their ongoing encouragement, editorial insights, and friendship are invaluable.

I'd like to thank my editor at Europa Editions, Kent Carroll, who has guided me through the completion of my last four books. He is a throwback to an era where editors paid attention to every word on a page. Once again, his concision and rigor allowed me to fine-tune the manuscript in a way that better enabled me to tell this story. Thanks, also, to Kent's assistant Raonaid Ryn and the entire team at Europa.

To my steadfast friends both living and gone who were with me through the events recounted in these pages I want to express profound gratitude. I treasure the way we continue to resonate in each other's lives.

Susan deserves a curtain call. It would not be an exaggeration to say her fortitude, courage, and love saved me. Had we not been married, I am not sure I would have survived long enough to write this book, or any other.

To the kingdom of tender colors.